Going Gluten Free

A Guide to Healthy Living, Dining, and Cooking

Yvonne M. Vissing, Ph.D.

Christopher Moore-Vissing, BA

Advance Praise for Going Gluten Free

Going Gluten Free is an outstanding resource, with magnificent tips on how to shop, cook, and enjoy healthy foods when living gluten free. Yvonne and Chris have lived it, and we are grateful they took time to write this book and share what they've learned.
—Douglas 'Duffy' MacKay, N.D.
Senior Vice President, Scientific and Regulatory Affairs
Council for Responsible Nutrition
www.crnusa.org

....

Going Gluten Free should be in the kitchen of anyone who has celiac disease. Vissing has done a remarkable job of collecting information most helpful to celiac patients, from diagnosis to eating out and setting up your gluten free kitchen. Readers will find this book is comprehensive, easy to read, and the recipes sound delicious. I look forward to recommending this book to my patients.
—Maria Larkin, M.Ed, RDN, LD
Better Gut Better Health Nutrition Counseling Services
http://www.bettergutbetterhealth.com/

....

Going Gluten Free is a thorough, practical primer on how to transition away from gluten in a safe and healthy manner. The gluten free diet presented in these pages is accurate and could also be called the gluten free lifestyle, because it covers so much more than food. This book covers how to set up your kitchen, safely dine out, travel, and enjoy a symptom-free life. Yvonne and Chris Vissing discuss all that, plus delicious recipes to get you started on the road to recovery.
—Christine Doherty, N.D.
New Hampshire
www.pointnatural.com

Yvonne Vissing's book *Going Gluten Free* is a must have for anyone newly diagnosed with gluten intolerance and for readers who want to eat, and feel, better. The book covers all aspects of celiac disease and the gluten free diet, including detailed information about dining out, shopping, cooking, health tips, and great gluten-free recipes.

—Scott Adams,
Celiac.com

A sophisticated and modern resource, *Going Gluten Free* is a valuable aid to sustaining a healthy gluten free lifestyle.

—Daniel Leffler, MD, MS
Director of Clinical Research
The Celiac Center at BIDMC
Director of QualityImprovement
Division of Gastroenterology
Beth Israel Deaconess Medical Center
Author of *Real Life with Celiac Disease*

Dedication

To Aunt Judy
from Chris

To Edna
from Yvonne

Contents

Foreword
Dr. Daniel Leffler

YOU ONLY HAVE TO diagnose one person with celiac disease to understand how significant this disorder is for patients, families, and their social circles. For decades the medical community underestimated the impact of a gluten free diet on the lives of people and families who live with celiac disease. And because this was a rare diagnosis, for the most part people struggled alone.

During the last few years, the United States has seen an explosion of progress in all facets of celiac disease, including scientific research, improved diagnosis, sophisticated patient support structures, and a gluten free section in virtually every supermarket. Yet, if anything, this increased awareness and understanding of celiac disease makes it increasingly clear how far we still have to go.

People with celiac disease still have frequent, ongoing, or intermittent symptoms, usually (but not always) related to inadvertent gluten exposure. For many adults the intestine fails to fully recover, and when healing does occur, it generally takes years. Extra-intestinal manifestations of celiac disease, including osteoporosis and neurological disorders, continue to be frequent and are often missed.

Finally, despite all the increased support and gluten free resources, patients with celiac disease still rate the difficulty of treatment higher than almost any other common medical disorder. Sophisticated and modern resources such as Going Gluten Free are valuable aids in sustaining a healthy gluten free lifestyle.

—Daniel Leffler, MD, MS
Director of Clinical Research
The Celiac Center at BIDMC
Director of Quality Improvement
Division of Gastroenterology
Beth Israel Deaconess Medical Center
Author of *Real Life With Celiac Disease*

Preface

EATING GOOD FOOD should be one of the greatest joys of our lives. Food is supposed to look and feel attractive, taste good, provide energy, and keep our bodies healthy. That's why it's so shocking to learn that grain—something we consume almost every day—can potentially make us sick. Approximately one in every 133 people in the United States has been diagnosed with gluten intolerance or celiac disease, a condition that causes our bodies to react badly after eating a protein found in wheat, barley, and rye.

But wheat and other grains are supposed to be good for us, aren't they?

In fact, grains aren't as wonderful as we once believed. Humans don't fully digest wheat, for example. Cows do fine with wheat because they have four stomachs, but wheat can be a challenge for us single-stomached humans. And for some people, the gluten found in grain is downright toxic.

The gluten free movement is among the fastest-growing nutritional trends in the world, even for people who don't have gluten sensitivity. For those with medical gluten issues, a 100 percent gluten free diet is the only existing treatment.

If you or someone you love has been diagnosed with gluten sensitivity or celiac disease

If you suspect your body isn't properly digesting gluten

If you want to change your diet and your lifestyle

. . . then keep reading this book!

Sure, going gluten free can be a challenge and it involves every aspect of your life, including how you eat, shop, dine out, your social life, and even a few emotional challenges. The good news is—you can solve this problem by yourself, without medication or expensive medical treatments. When you learn how to take control of your diet, the benefits can be quick and amazing.

Ten years ago when Chris, the co-author of this book, realized he had every symptom of celiac disease, we decided to give the gluten free diet a try. At the time, this was easier said than done. No manuals or books were on the market, so like many things in life, we did it the hard way thinking it was the easy way. We bought gluten free products and tried to work them into our typical diet. This didn't work nearly as well as we expected. The result? Living gluten free doomed us to eating slimy, cardboard-like, tasteless food that killed our appetites. We knew there had to be a better way and we went in search of it.

Through trial and error we've come to understand that being gluten free is actually easy, not more expensive, and absolutely delicious as well as healthy. With unabashed pride we confidently announce we have become gourmet gluten free cooks. People love coming to our house and even wheat-eaters want me to cook gluten free (GF) for them because the food tastes so good. But this result didn't come overnight. It took years to figure out.

That's why we want to share what we learned, so you'll have an easier time and will love being gluten free right from the start. The pages that follow will chronicle the journey to becoming gluten free and happy. Here's what you'll learn:

Shopping Gluten Free

In the beginning we spent a lot of money on products we ended up tossing out. We had no idea what to buy or how to shop, because we didn't know how to make the transition to gluten free cooking. Gluten free products tend to be expensive and you can waste a lot of money buying things you wouldn't feed a dog. We'll help you figure out what products to pick up for one time use and what staples you'll need to keep on-hand.

In theory, shopping should be easy, because grocery stores now feature gluten free products in their health food aisles. Just stock up on these and throw everything else away, right?

Not so fast! A label that says "gluten free" doesn't mean a product is healthier; some of these foods are highly processed and filled with chemicals. Besides that, a product labeled "wheat free" may not be gluten free, and even food marked gluten free may not be safe for people with celiac disease. In Chapter Two, we'll help you sort out these confusing labels.

The Gluten Free Kitchen

We will talk frankly about kitchens in this book, and not the type used by Top Chef or Julia Child. We're talking about normal kitchens. You may not realize it yet, but even the tiny amount of gluten in a few bread crumbs can lead to excruciating symptoms, especially for someone with celiac disease.

If you're serious about going gluten free you will need to restructure your kitchen, which means taking stock of the cooking areas—microwave, stovetop, and oven, items like fryers and waffle irons, as well as preparation areas, food storage areas, and dish cleaning areas. We'll show you how in Chapter Three.

Yvonne M. Vissing, Ph.D.
Christopher Moore-Vissing, BA

How to Cook Gluten Free

Maybe your idea of gourmet cooking involves a can opener, a freezer, or a microwave oven. Or perhaps you have specialty dishes you love to prepare—things you're famous for cooking. I found that substituting items into my old cooking style and recipes was a hit-or-miss proposition. Some recipes worked well, but others flopped. Expanding my recipe repertoire was important in becoming a gourmet gluten free cook. Now I've figured out how to fix delicious, easy, and cost-effective gluten free food, and I'm giving you my favorite secrets and recipes in Chapter Six.

Dining Out

During our journey to becoming gluten free we came to realize that *we* were making the process unnecessarily hard. *We* were the biggest obstacles to enjoying a gluten free lifestyle. Understanding our relationship with food and those who feed us is an important aspect of the dining experience. We will show you how to make every-day eating at home a healthy and delicious experience. We'll also talk candidly about dining out and give you suggestions on how to make sure you don't get sick.

Going out to eat is far from simple when you're gluten free. Just because a restaurant advertises itself as gluten free doesn't mean it is. In Chapter Five and Appendix A, we'll show you what to look for and offer tips about the safest places to eat, along with ideas about how to order and what to question or avoid.

Attitude is Everything

We've found you can't expect others to be as attentive to gluten free issues as you are. How we deal with others and educate them is important. This means being assertive and asking key questions to make sure you eat safely. Whether you're going to an amusement park, a wedding reception, or having a quick lunch at the office cafeteria, we're here to help you have a pleasant dining experience.

This book starts by looking at what gluten is and why people want to go gluten free. It ends by giving you a crash course on how to become gluten free and love it. We hope to help you to realize that going gluten free can be a positive change to your life.

Chris never gets sick when we cook our gourmet gluten free foods at home. More restaurants are being attentive to the details of gluten free dining, but there are still black holes to fall into that can make life unnecessarily difficult. Carry this book when you travel, when you shop, and keep it handy in the kitchen.

We hope *Going Gluten Free* will be a valuable road map on your journey to gluten freedom.

Chapter 1
Going Gluten Free

GOING GLUTEN FREE is becoming more commonplace, even vogue, in our culture. While celebrities may announce they're gluten free because they're following a fashionable trend, most people who become gluten free would prefer not to.

Chris would give anything to have a burger on a real bun. He'd love to chow down on Oreo ice cream, oatmeal cookies with dried cranberries, or graham cracker s'mores. But he can't, because those foods aren't safe for him.

He'd love not to read the ingredient list on every product before he decides whether he can eat it. While he appreciates gluten free pastas so he can have macaroni-and-cheese, and gluten free flour for home-made bread, frankly they're just not the same. He'd be so happy to order a gluten free pizza that doesn't taste like cardboard or go out with the rest of the family for dinner and order anything on the menu. He'd like to not second guess whether the cook in the restaurant knew enough not to fry the eggs on the same surface they made French toast.

Going gluten free isn't a choice for most people. It's a health necessity.

What is Gluten?

Glutens are elastic proteins that help bread rise and allow foods to maintain their shape. They're also used as thickening agents in a variety of products seemingly unrelated to bread type foods. Glutens are most commonly found in grains such as wheat, barley, and rye.

Oats don't have gluten, but the usual consensus is to stay away from them unless they're certified to be gluten free. Oat and wheat are often grown in fields adjacent to one another, processed in the same grain elevators, milled with the same equipment, or transported in containers that haven't been scrubbed in between shipments. This often leads to cross-contamination between the two grains, and as a result oats often aren't safe. If oats are grown and processed in certified gluten free conditions, then they may be safe—but it's hard to know for sure. That's why gluten free foods labeled "processed in a facility that also processes wheat products" can be dangerous.

Gluten hides everywhere. I was excited to bring home a pack of Newman's Own wheat-free Fig Newtons until Chris read the label and found barley, a gluten, in the list of ingredients. I got suckered by thinking wheat-free meant gluten free.

A variety of additives, such as monosodium glutamate, may contain gluten, or gluten may be disguised food starch—which could be corn (which is safe and not a gluten based protein) or wheat, which is a major problem for people with gluten intolerance.

Gluten is found mainly in food, but also sneaks into everyday products such as medicine, vitamins, lip balm, and even certain drinks. The malt in beer and other products is usually made from barley, which contains gluten. Gluten is everywhere, and when you go gluten free you can't take anything for granted.

Why Is Gluten Such an Issue Now?

We've been taught that whole grain products are healthy and wholesome. The old food pyramid emphasized grain for fiber and nutrients, although we can get the same benefits from other foods.

More gluten based products are consumed in the world today than ever before—and as gluten consumption increases, so do the health problems associated with it. The human digestive system doesn't fully digest wheat. This can lead to a wide array of issues with our bodies.

Anthropologists know wheat was grown as far back as 9000 B.C. However, most people didn't consume large amounts of grain, because it had to be cracked open, ground by hand, sifted, and then cooked. This involved process was challenging to accomplish with primitive culinary tools. Moreover, whole grains had a tendency to spoil quickly and eating food made with rancid grain could make people sick. For instance, a bad rye crop has been associated with the creation of the Salem Witch Trials when an ergot fungus on the rye may have been responsible for the hallucinations and problems alleged by those possessed by "witches" (Dean 2012).

Over time people discovered that if they stripped the germ away from the bran in a process called milling, the grain could be transformed into soft white flour and kept longer. Inventions such as the reaper, the steel plow, and high speed steel roller mills, helped produce larger amounts of the fine white flour. The demand for white instead of brown flour increased because it tasted better and created fluffier food products. As railroads crossed the nation, transportation of goods made flour more available and affordable. Soon, the masses had access to refined wheat flour that was once a luxury item for the wealthy.

The wheat we use today is different from 100 years ago—more refined, and containing more gluten. Soft wheat varieties were commonly used in the United States until around 1870, when varieties of hard spring wheat from Central Europe were introduced into the marketplace. These wheat types contained higher protein or gluten contents and were more desirable because they resulted in lighter bread and flakier baked goods. For instance, the Puritans with their hearty wheat bread could never have baked the elegant and delicious croissant.

Wheat was the basis for a whole new set of food items. During the late 1890s Quaker, Kellogg, and Post cereal companies began developing breakfast cereals that used wheat products—shredded wheat, wheat flakes, Chex, Grape Nuts, and Cream of Wheat. During the 1930s, Kraft introduced macaroni and cheese dinners. When meat was hard to procure during wartime, people were encouraged to stretch it by adding cracker crumbs or other wheat products as breading, or for meat loaf.

During the 1970s the medical community targeted heart disease and cholesterol, telling us whole wheat was a healthy dietary option. When the fast food industry came on the scene, wheat was the basis for burgers, pizza, and bagels. Wheat is now the most cultivated of any crop worldwide—and it's also associated with a large variety of physical and mental health problems.

Here's the problem in a nutshell: We're overloading our bodies with products the human digestive system wasn't meant to deal with. Our diet changed over the millenniums, but our bodies did not. And to complicate matters, the symptoms of gluten intolerance are so diverse, we may not recognize them at first.

Types of Gluten Intolerance and Celiac Disease

Some people say they have a gluten allergy, but it's important to know this isn't an allergy in the true sense of the word. People who have gluten intolerance, sensitivity, or celiac disease experience adverse symptoms that may seem like allergies on the surface, but are actually autoimmune disorders.

Think of gluten problems as a spectrum, with allergic symptoms on the low end, sensitivity and intolerance to gluten in the middle range, and finally, celiac disease.

Allergy-type symptoms Sensitivity and Intolerance Celiac Disease

Gluten intolerance and sensitivity

These terms are often used interchangeably to describe health problems associated with gluten. Basically, this means your body doesn't react well to foods containing gluten and you should avoid them. Often, the lines between gluten intolerance, sensitivity, and celiac disease are fuzzy. In fact, people in the medical community don't agree on the protocol for identifying these issues.

- Some patients are misdiagnosed, either through faulty testing or inconclusive results.
- Other people start with gluten intolerance and later "graduate" to celiac disease.
- Still others feel better with a gluten free diet and never move on to celiac disease.

This unpleasant disorder was first diagnosed in the United Kingdom back in the late 1980s. Historical records indicate that President John F. Kennedy frequently suffered from a gastro-intestinal disorder—probably gluten intolerance.[1] That makes sense, because gluten issues are more common among people of Celtic background.

While some people believe intolerance and sensitivity are emotional problems, those with gluten issues know it isn't just in their heads. The symptoms are similar (but usually less severe) than celiac disease, and may include everything from gastric misery to skin irritation, depression, and emotional distress. Even the symptoms of autism can be related to gluten intolerance.[2]

The main difference among gluten problems is that people who are intolerant or sensitive to gluten have not (yet) developed leaky intestinal walls, as is common in celiac patients. Symptoms are usually less pronounced with intolerance and sensitivity. Controlling your diet by going gluten free diet may keep you from developing celiac disease.

---

1   Gluten free Standards Association 2011
2   Fran Lowry. Gluten Sensitivity to Autism. Medscape Medical News. (July 5, 2013). http://bit.ly/1DkXIMg

Celiac disease

Celiac is the most severe form of gluten intolerance, and even products mildly contaminated with gluten can lead to distressing symptoms. Celiac victims experience an auto-immune disorder in which the lining of the small intestine (villi) is damaged and nutrients can't be absorbed. Celiac disease is also known as:

- celiac sprue,
- nontropical sprue, and
- gluten-sensitive enteropathy.

This distressing illness affects nearly three million people in the United States, although an estimated 97 percent of celiac sufferers are undiagnosed.[3] Unfortunately, this disease tends to run in families. The good news is—you can be tested for some of these auto-immune genes by using a swabbed sample from the inside of your mouth. A home-testing kit is available online.[4] Having the genetic markers in your family does not mean you'll develop celiac disease, but your risk factors are higher.

The other good news is: this disease is fully treatable by diet alone.

Celiac disease may be something you've had since childhood, or it can be triggered by an event that stresses your body, such as surgery, pregnancy, physical injury, illness, or emotional trauma.

When your gut doesn't properly digest glutens, the undigested protein triggers what seems to be a toxic immune response. Toxins and fragments of gluten enter the bloodstream through the intestinal wall, in what is known as *leaky gut syndrome*.[5] If you have celiac disease, your body identifies these fragments as invaders. The immune system launches an all-out attack against your own body. Your immune system targets the lining of the small intestine, causing the villi (hairlike projections) to flatten, which affects their ability to

---

3   Fasano et al 2003
4   EnteroLabs at https://www.enterolab.com/
5   Leaky gut syndrome leads to many disorders besides celiac disease.

digest and absorb nutrients in the food. When people have difficulty absorbing nutrients, malabsorption may leave them anemic, tired, and weak. You can eat plenty of good food and maintain a healthy diet, yet still be malnourished.

Symptoms of Gluten Intolerance and Celiac Disease

The symptoms of people with gluten problems may seem bewildering because they can affect the entire body. This plague of seemingly unrelated problems may cause misery in our lives, but seem unrelated at first. That makes gluten intolerance difficult to diagnose and easy to confuse with other diseases. Plus, it isn't picked up with traditional medical tests your doctor routinely orders.

Who would think a single disease could link digestive disorders, nausea, stomach pain, diarrhea, skin rashes, seborrhea, anemia, chronic fatigue, neurological problems, migraine headaches and depression into a single syndrome that's food related? If you have a "gut feeling" that gluten in an issue in your life and want to look at the signs and symptoms, I'll break them into categories.

Gastrointestinal troubles

These are the classic symptoms of gluten problems within your body, but they aren't always the most common signs. Remember, your entire body gets involved because the immune system is running amuck.

- Abdominal pain and distension
- Acid reflux
- Bloating
- Constipation
- Diarrhea
- Gas and flatulence
- Greasy, foul-smelling stools that float

- Nausea
- Vomiting
- Weight loss or gain

You may know people with celiac disease who are thin and emaciated, but that isn't always the case. Some people gain weight and become obese.

Extra-intestinal symptoms

Symptoms that don't directly involve the gastric tract are known as extra-intestinal. This list of symptoms is so diverse that the list tops over 250, which shows how important the small intestine's job is to our well-being—and how the immune system can manifest itself. Here are some of the most common symptoms:

- Iron deficiency leading to fatigue and weakness
- Mineral and vitamin deficiencies
- Joint or bone pain
- Headaches, including migraines
- Poor concentration
- Infertility
- Abnormal menstrual cycles
- Nerve damage, called peripheral neuropathy
- Dental enamel deficiencies
- Seizures
- Respiratory problems
- Cancer sores
- Lactose intolerance
- Eczema, psoriasis, rosacea, acne, and other skin conditions
- Autoimmune disorders such as lupus erythematosus, Hashimoto's disease, Sjögren's syndrome, and others
- Osteoporosis
- Hair loss
- Bruising

- Low blood sugar (hypoglycemia)
- Muscle cramping
- Nosebleeds
- Swelling and inflammation
- Night blindness

As I mentioned earlier, celiac disease has also been linked to other discoreders. Infertility and abnormally slow growth of a fetus are other issues you wouldn't normally think to associate with intestinal disease, but they can also be related to gluten intolerance.

Gluten intolerance and celiac disease affect people of all ages, though symptoms may manifest differently in children. In women iron deficiencies may interfere with pregnancy and can result in low birth weight infants or miscarriage. In hopes of preventing celiac disease, breastfeeding and delaying the introduction of foods containing gluten until after four months is suggested to help children avoid exposure to gluten before their bodies have fully developed. Undiagnosed gluten problems in babies may prove to be life-threatening, and the most common signs include chronic diarrhea, distended abdomen, and difficulties gaining weight and growing.

For older children, malabsorption of nutrients can be detrimental to normal growth and development, resulting in problems such as delayed growth and short stature, delayed puberty, and dental enamel defects of the permanent teeth. Chris has a cousin with celiac disease who was small for his age. It's curious that in siblings with the same biological parents, one may have gluten reactions while the other does not. This is the genetic luck of the draw, and is another reason most people don't realize they have gluten issues until later in life.

As people grow older, new symptoms may appear, or the old symptoms become chronic. Tiredness, irritability, weakness, bone pain, ulcers in the mouth, skin irritations (often on the elbows, knees or scalp), headaches, depression, and anxiety may rise to the point of being debilitating.

There is some concern that in extreme cases, celiac disease may be related to severe psychological problems that can lead to suicidal ideation or attempts if left untreated. Lillian, a girl of Irish background and the first person I knew of who had celiac disease, was diagnosed with depression and tried to commit suicide. Since then, we've learned of many celiac people who express anxiety, depression, and suicidal ideation. Therefore, it's important to remember that behavior which seems totally unrelated to gluten may actually have a huge correlation.

Celiac disease is thought to be associated with other conditions, including:

- Type 1, or insulin-dependent diabetes
- Autoimmune thyroid disease
- Ulcers and colitis
- Autoimmune liver disease
- Rheumatoid arthritis
- Addison's disease
- Sjögren's syndrome, a condition in which the glands that produce tears and saliva are affected.
- Dermatitis herpetiformis, an itchy, blistering skin disorder that may occur when gluten is ingested.[6]

If a person with celiac disease continues to eat gluten, studies show an increased chance for developing gastrointestinal cancer, perhaps a by a factor of 40 to 100 times that of the normal population.

Diagnosing Gluten Intolerance and Celiac Disease

Like many other people, we self-diagnosed celiac disease for Chris. We didn't realize this illness ran on his father's side of the family. His Northern European grandmother had health problems that were evidently gluten related, but that was before people commonly understood gluten issues. His father's generation apparently escaped celiac disease (it often skips a generation), but Chris and his first

6   (Heathy villi 2014)

cousin did not escape. When Chris visited his cousin while in his mid-20's, he discovered they had similar health issues. I wish we'd known sooner. Even when Chris was a child we talked with doctors about his various symptoms. None of them had linked his problems together as a sign of celiac disease. After the fact, one sighed and said, "Wow, I should have seen that."

Yes—but at least we know now. And knowing has changed one of the most fundamental aspects of life—how and what we eat.

We've also been forced to learn more about biology, physiology, nutrition, and health issues than we ever expected to know. Learning how our bodies work is not a bad thing. Going gluten free meant rolling up our sleeves to dig into information and find out more about this pervasive health problem. Some health care practitioners are helpful, but we learned that going gluten free puts you on a course of self-advocacy.

Like Chris, many people diagnose themselves after learning about the symptoms from a family member, friends, or the media. Eliminating gluten from the diet and watching your body's reaction is a great way to test yourself.

This condition is often missed by physicians, although awareness is on the rise. In too many cases, patients are treated for the varied symptoms of gluten intolerance without ever finding the underlying cause. This can involve taking multiple drugs and undergoing expensive treatments that never touch the real issue—gluten.

An endoscopy of the small intestine *with a biopsy* is the gold standard for a medical diagnosis, along with a series of five blood tests for antibodies associated with the disease: EMA anti-endomysial antibody), tTGIgA or anti-tissue transglutaminase antibody, anti DGP for people with an IgA deficiency. The blood tests will only be accurate if you're eating gluten.

A company called EnteroLab has developed a home stool test for gluten sensitivity and other gastro intestinal conditions. This test in noninvasive and doesn't require a doctor's order, but you will probably have to pay for it yourself.[7]

Genetic testing can be done with blood, stool, or a new saliva home-testing kit. This will show whether or not you have the genes associated with celiac disease.[8]

Managing Gluten Intolerance and Celiac Disease

I'll state the good news again: You can control and treat these disorders yourself without drugs or medical treatments. You need to eliminate gluten from your diet. That's it. Continue reading this book and you'll learn how a gluten free diet can be nutritious, delicious, and healthy. Intestinal healing may take a while, but if you start now you can begin rejuvenating your health and your lifestyle.

You can't prevent gluten issues, but you can learn to manage them. In rare cases, people have had the disease for such a long time that their intestines are unable to heal, and they may suffer from refractory celiac disease that doesn't respond even to dietary changes.

Since awareness of celiac disease and gluten intolerance is relatively recent, a huge number people have lived for many, many years feeling bad and not knowing they had the disease. For sensitive people who've spent a lifetime eating gluten, the older they get, the greater the likelihood of intestinal damage.

Scientists continue looking for factors associated with who develops celiac disease. This includes the length of time a person was breastfed, the age a person started eating gluten-containing foods, and the amount of gluten-containing foods one eats. Some studies indicate the longer a person was breastfed, the later the symptoms of celiac disease appear.[9]

7   http://bit.ly/1kxSpFG
8   American Clinical Board of Nutrition Dr. Peter Osborne's Gluten Sensitivity vs Celiac Disease vs Gluten Intolerance http://bit.ly/1BKPFbr, http://bit.ly/1EtNsHG, and http://bit.ly/1yuh2Fp
9   Jean Guest. Breastfeeding and Celiac Disease. Lifeline. Winter 2004, vol xxiv, no 1: 22-24. http://bit.ly/1Ez5cj9

Who Gets Celiac Disease?

Celiac disease and gluten sensitivities appear to affect men and women equally. It was once thought to affect only children, but today is commonly diagnosed in people between the ages of 30 and 45. People with European or Anglo-Celtic ancestry seem more predisposed to non-celiac gluten sensitivity and celiac disease than others. Sometimes this is referred to as an Irish disease, with a rate in Ireland of one in 100 people afflicted. In the United Kingdom, the reported rates vary from one in 100 to one in 300 people. In Italy, one in 250 people seem to have gluten intolerance. Data indicates that people from the Punjab region of India, Pakistan, and the Middle East also experience higher levels of gluten intolerance. Recent studies show it affects Hispanic, Black, and Asian populations as well. In the United States, current rates of people with gluten intolerance are projected as one in 133 people. This is higher than many other mainstream diseases—yet only recently has this illness made the news.

Data indicates gluten intolerance seems to run in families, with about ten percent of the immediate family affected. Often, gluten intolerance is apparent in every age group within a family, or it may skip generations. Some scientists feel the predisposition for gluten intolerance is there even when family members don't experience observable symptoms.

Some researchers suggest that 10 to 15 percent of the population has some form of gluten intolerance, but most of these people either have no digestive-tract symptoms or mild symptoms.

Gluten Free Resources: The Devil is in the Details

We discovered that most doctors don't know much about celiac disease, gluten intolerance, or going gluten free. None of our doctors diagnosed Chris until he put two and two together. If you've read this far, you already know celiac is a sneaky disease and challenging to diagnose, especially in the early stages.

Most doctors tried to be helpful by giving us superficial instructions such as "keep away from gluten" without proving details. And with gluten, "the devil's in the details," as the old saying goes. Yes, we know not to eat a burger from McDonalds because the bun is not gluten free. But are the burgers 100 percent meat? Are the seasonings safe? Are they cooked without cross-contamination? Gluten is everywhere, and you need to become a private-eye in order to find it.

We found great information and support from social networking sites. When in doubt over whether a food is safe, we go to **Celiac. com** and ask. Usually we find a reliable answer. This is a wonderful thing! We've used this website while standing in the aisle looking at products in the grocery store. We use it in restaurants to learn what people have to say about particular menu items, or when trying to find out about what type of corned beef we should serve at our St. Patrick's Day party.

Celiac Disease and Gluten Intolerance Websites:

- Celiac.com (http://www.celiac.com) is the premier website for people with Celiac disease and gluten intolerance. This marvelous website is rich with information about all gluten issues.
- The National Digestive Diseases Information Clearinghouse (NDDIC), which is a service of the National Institute of Diabetes and Digestive and Kidney Diseases (NIDDK), National Institutes of Health (NIH), provides a variety of information and links that may be helpful. Go to: http://1. usa.gov/UzlFA0
- The Healthy Villi is a newsletter and organization that hosts annual conferences and a variety of educational and support events for the celiac community. (www.healthyvilli. org). It recently changed to NECO—New England Celiac Organization—but their information is useful for people everywhere.

- The Gluten Syndrome (http://www.theglutensyndrome.net/) is a website focusing on patient perspectives for living a gluten free lifestyle. This site references a variety of medical and practical information and resources.
- Gluten Free Faces is a social networking site that links people with others who have gluten issues. It provides information on health, products, restaurants, and it is full of super information. Find it at (http://www.glutenfreefaces.com).
- This gluten free message board has 32,000 members and 559,000 posts. Visit celiacdiseaseforum/messageboard
- The Celiac Diva (www.theceliacdiva.com) provides a younger-audience approach to celiac disease and the issue of gluten intolerance. It provides links to products (such as gluten free nail polish and cosmetics), science links, resources, and opportunities to network.

Other useful websites:

American Celiac Disease Alliance www.americanceliac.org

Celiac Sprue Association http://www.csaceliacs.org

Celiac Disease Foundation www.celiac.org

Celiac Disease and Gluten Free Diet Information
http://www.celiac.com/

Celiac Support Organizations
http://www.csaceliacs.org/celiac_centers.jsp

Defeat The Wheat http://defeatthewheat.com

Gluten Intolerance Group www.gluten.net

National Foundation for Celiac Awareness
www.celiaccentral.org

Celiac Center www.celiaccenter.org

Gluten Free Dietitian www.glutenfreedietitian.com

Gluten Free Diet www.glutenfreediet.ca

Delete The Wheat www.deletethewheat.com

New England Celiac society www.celiacnow.org

University of Maryland Center for Celiac Research
http://medschool.umaryland.edu/celiac/

Children's Hospital Boston http://bit.ly/1bLkrec

Gluten Free Restaurant Awareness Program
http://www.glutenfreerestaurants.org

Celiac Disease Center at Columbia University, New York City
http://www.celiacdiseasecenter.columbia.edu/celiac-disease

Celiac medical centers

We love our family doctors, but frankly, they don't know that much about celiac or gluten free issues. So we made an appointment at the celiac program at Beth Israel Deaconess Hospital in Boston and worked with national celiac expert Dr. Daniel Leffler, a researcher and author on the topic. He understands the physical, social, nutritional, and emotional dynamics of celiac disorders. Going to someone who "gets it" is important when you search for a doctor. On several occasions Dr. Leffler helped Chris figure out what's going on inside his gut and how to manage better.

Several specialized celiac and gluten intolerance medical centers are scattered around the country, and more are emerging as the problem increases. They all provide helpful information about gluten and can work with individuals, organizations, and restaurants to ensure gluten issues are adequately addressed. Some of the major celiac medical centers include:

Baltimore MD: Celiac Center at the University of Maryland Medical Center. Dr. Alessio Fasano is the director and one of the country's experts on Celiac disease. Check out his books. http://umm.edu/health/medical/altmed/condition/celiac-sprue

Bloomington MN. Celiac Center of Minnesota. http://bit.ly/1Cr2MkJ

Boston MA: Celiac Center at Beth Israel Deaconess Medical Center. Director, Dr. Ciaran Kelly and Dr. Daniel Leffler (co-author of Real Life With Celiac Disease). We have found them to be extraordinarily helpful. http://www.bidmc.org/celiaccenter

Chicago IL: Celiac Disease Center at the University of Chicago Medical Center. http://bit.ly/1ae1IHU

Knoxville, TN: Celiac Center at the University of Tennessee Medical Center. http://bit.ly/1G2Z5Wj

Livingston, NJ: Kogan Celiac Center at the Barnabas Health Center. http://bit.ly/1BLEYph

New York, NY: Celiac Center at Columbia University Medical Center. Dr. Peter H. R. Green is the director. http://bit.ly/1mGwuHZ

Philadelphia, PA. Celiac Center at Thomas Jefferson University Hospital. http://www.jeffersonhospital.org/departments-and-services/celiac-center.aspx

Philadelphia PA. Center for Celiac Disease. Children's Hospital of Philadelphia. http://bit.ly/1Nyx2x6

San Diego CA: William K. Warren Medical Research Center for Celiac Disease. University of California at San Diego Medical Center. http://bit.ly/1GIm3kN

Stanford CA. Celiac Sprue Clinic. Stanford University Medical Center. https://stanfordhealthcare.org/

The list of resources for people with gluten issues is vast and I've only listed the major ones. Please feel free to contact us if you find new sources. Everyone benefits from sharing information and networking.

Putting it All Together

Going gluten free is more than a fad for health-freaks. It's a healthy dietary and culinary trend that's here to stay, and gluten free dining is already main stream in many parts of the world. Cutting wheat and gluten from the diet is a choice for some people. But for those who have gluten intolerance on celiac disease, there is no choice. People with celiac disease work hard to stay healthy and avoid a wide variety of physical and mental health problems. Glutening them is the same as poisoning them; they may not die from it, but they feel awful. You can do long term damage by not being sensitive to their needs.

It's important to be educated on this topic, no matter who you are. I'm willing to bet you know people who are gluten free, even if they haven't told you. Once you become aware, you'll blink in amazement at how many people have gluten issues.

If you're someone who needs a gluten free diet, the great thing is—once you learn how to go gluten free it doesn't have to be a big deal. In fact, it can be easy.

Chapter 2
Shopping Gluten Free

IT DOESN'T TAKE a rocket scientist to recognize the trend toward more gluten free products on the market. Only a few years ago when Chris was first diagnosed with celiac disease, we found only a few GF products and brands on the shelves—and none of these were tempting. It was "slim pickins" to say the least. Now you'll easily find an array of GF soup, meats, cookies, crackers, breads, pastas, grains, and processed foods. Some of these GF items are far superior to their traditional glutened counterparts. However, the selection depends upon where you live and where you shop. We live in New England and have little problem finding GF foods, but when we travel in the Midwest, it's another story. The GF foods are there, but much harder to find and choices are limited. Eating GF in my Indiana home town is challenging at best. Eating in Denver, for example, is great, because GF food and savvy servers seems to be a normal, expected, and standard experience. Where you live colors how easy or hard going gluten free can be.

If you live in a community where resources are hard to find, you can still go gluten free without issue—it will just take planning ahead and proactive decision making. The change in your diet may also mean shopping online and having products shipped to you, or going on shopping sprees to the big city where you can stock up on staple ingredients.

When you do a computer search, the results clearly show gluten free shopping and dining are major concerns for the general public. A recent Google search showed over 88 million hits for the term "gluten free." According to the Gluten free.com website, information on gluten free eating has doubled in recent years. Gluten free food isn't a niche market anymore; it is becoming part of the mainstream and is here to stay.

The Changing Face of Food Production and Labeling

Unless you live on a farm and grow your own food or shop at local farmer's markets, chances are you're shopping in the large grocery store chains. Authors like Marion Nestle (2013) have written about food safety and food politics, what to eat and what to avoid, and how to shop for the healthiest foods. The issue of food contamination and changes in the food industry are usually credited back to Rachel Carson's environmental and food impact manifesto of the *Silent Spring* back in 1962. My grandparents were farmers, my mama was a farm girl who lived in the city and kept true to her rural culinary roots, and I'm a product of the organic food days. We have never had a plethora of processed foods around, yet admittedly we compromised our back-to-the-roots background one Coke, one Oreo, and one serving of McDonalds fries at a time.

For a while during the transition from plain whole foods to processed products, we had no laws for ingredient labeling. The Food and Drug Administration either didn't exist or lacked the authority to enforce standards. The lack of transparency in food labeling was a problem for people who thought they were eating one food, only to find it was contaminated with another, like people with penicillin allergies who became ill after eating poultry shot up with antibiotics.

Red dye became an additive issue in the 1960s when it was allegedly associated with cancer. The "sugar blues" movement came about in the 1970s when consumption of sugar was associated with a variety of emotional and health problems. Then there was the peanut allergy movement that led to peanut butter no longer being considered a safe staple for kids. One by one, processed product concerns have elevated different issues that eventually made all additives and processing procedures more transparent for consumers.

This is a blessing for people who have celiac disease or gluten sensitivities. According to the Gluten free Standards Association, gluten free and other food testing groups are popping up everywhere. Learn more about these groups on page 179.

The general rule of thumb is—the fresher and more unprocessed a food is, the greater the chance it is gluten free. Conversely, the more processed a food is, the higher the risk of it containing gluten or being contaminated by gluten.

General Shopping Observations

The fact is, many gluten free foods are not marked that way. Most fresh fruits, vegetables, meats, and dairy products are GF and safe. This is the mantra of the natural foods people. Less processing usually equals healthier food. The more natural and in a whole, original state the food is, the better the chance it is safe. Isn't that a simple guideline to follow?

Food processors are now required by law to list ingredients. Food allergens, including gluten, must be on the label. That is a comfort! Sometimes the ingredients are listed in teeny fonts that make them hard to read while standing in the grocery aisles. I recommend carrying a small magnifying glass. Or, if you have a smart phone, you can easily check product ingredients on site.

Foods that ought to be safe but are processed in factories that also process wheat may be contaminated. If someone has a serious reaction to gluten, these should-have-been-safe foods are dangerous. For instance, nuts should normally be safe. But read the cans —some nuts are processed in facilities that also process wheat. If you're buying plain nuts, that should be fine, but they could be exposed to gluten on machines that put a tasty coating on some varieties of nuts. Wheat can accidentally cling to the now not-safe nuts. Tempting as it may be to purchase delicious looking items that read "made in a facility that also processes wheat," don't do it. You'll be gambling. Is it worth the risk?

Then there's the grey zone, where foods like oats are sometimes safe and sometimes not, depending on where they were grown. If they were harvested next to a wheat field—guess what? Those oats are not gluten free.

Because some products are actually gluten free but haven't received certification from GF organizations, we've become adept at reading product ingredients. Often we're able to find great products that are safe, but aren't marked GF. We now know what ingredients to look for. Knowing which companies have dedicated their products to be GF is also helpful because it means if we're in a rush, the probability of grabbing a safe product is high. For instance, we know Frank's Red Hot sauce is safe; so is their Sweet Chili sauce. Recently at the store I plopped two bottles of their Buffalo Wings sauce into my cart without reading the ingredients until I got home, because I know their products are usually GF. Reading the label, it looked safe, but I couldn't find an actual gluten free statement on the bottle. So I went to the Celiac.com website and found, sure enough, it was listed as gluten free. While it may take a smidge more effort to make certain a product is safe, that's a lot better than to risk making someone deathly ill.

Going gluten free means we have to take a hard look at our dietary choices. Processed foods are often delicious, we agree. They also contain lots of fat, salt, sugar, and other magical ingredients that make them taste so good that we want another chip, another cookie, another bite, or another portion. Plain and "honest" corn, meat, rice, or vegetables may be better for us, but we sometimes long for ways to cook them with more pizzazz. This means if we want them to be tasty, we have to know our friendly condiments and seasonings, and use recipes that enhance their goodness. Eating should be fun as well as healthy, and therein lies much of the challenge of gluten free cooking. Once you get it down, this isn't a big deal. But if you've been addicted to processed foods and fast food, it may take a bit of adjustment until you're in the swing of gluten free.

Where to Shop Gluten Free

Naturally, where you shop for gluten free products will largely depend upon where you live. For instance, stores that promote natural and organic foods (like Whole Foods or health food stores) have a higher probability of stocking GF products than convenience stores, which tend to sell more processed foods. It's frankly hard to find GF products at small stores like the Circle K or 7-11, although they sell a variety of must-have products.

I used to shop at several stores that specialized in carrying gluten free products. But many of them charged exorbitant prices, which led me to cook in a way that reserved the gluten free only for Chris. He got the corn pasta while the rest of us ate the wheat. We did this because it was cost effective, but it alienated him, made him feel different, and impacted our family eating experience. Today, many of these GF specialty stores have gone out of business because mainstream groceries are carrying more gluten free and natural food products. As I shopped in the going out of business sale at My Low Carb Life in Peabody, Massachusetts, the manager was sad because, while gluten free foods were more in demand, fewer people shopped at her store. The reason for the shift was simple—the local big-box grocery stores saw a growing market of shoppers who purchased gluten free items and they started carrying more types and brands at lower prices.

Today, gluten free cookies, crackers, breads, cakes, pastas, and mixes and products of all kinds can be found in traditional grocery stores. Betty Crocker gluten free brownie mix may sit on the shelf right beside her wheat variety. This makes shopping a lot more convenient for the patrons.

However, grocery stores carry what sells—and depending on where you live, gluten free products may not be fast-movers, as compared with glutened foods. This means selections may be limited in your town, although I can buy over 80 percent of my gluten free items at local grocery stores. When you need a product and can't find it locally, online shopping and shipping is a great alternative. I'll talk more about the best GF shopping websites in a minute.

Food availability is an issue because it dictates what will be served. Running here, there, and everywhere to find a particular product is time consuming, and sometimes we never find the item we're looking for. This means creating substitutions or making an entirely different dish.

Chris's godmother Fran in Alaska sends him boxes of delicious GF products we've never seen in New England. She finds processed GF products that are tasty and healthy, from soup to scones. Even with these regional differences, cooks everywhere can now make fantastic gluten free dishes.

Foods Ingredients: What's Safe and What Isn't

The most obvious way to manage celiac disease and gluten intolerance is not to eat anything with gluten in it. That sounds easy, doesn't it?

Unfortunately, it's far more complicated than regular people expect, until they figure out the system. Once you make the commitment to following a gluten free diet, there are plenty of helpful sources. For example, the website www.Celiac.com offers a search engine that enables you to enter a particular type of food, or even a certain brand, and find out if it's safe. You can also find a detailed list of safe gluten free products and manufacturers by going to the Gluten free Certification Organization website: http://www.gfco.org/.

As you begin going gluten free, it seems gluten is hidden in everything you want to eat. That's partly because most of us are accustomed to eating processed foods and wheat based products. Our first reaction is to continue eating the same way, but substitute non-wheat products. While that strategy works for some people, a better option is to change the way you approach eating and meal planning.

The new approach begins when you realign your thinking: Instead of creating gluten free menus you hope will be satisfying, instead create healthy and delicious menus that happen to be gluten free. This wording demonstrates a fundamental shift in perception. Basically, a diet that's richer in natural foods is a good starting place for everyone, gluten free or not. As a general rule, natural and simple foods are better for everyone.

Vegetables are always safe; boiled, baked, steamed, sautéed, and raw. They only become dangerous for someone with gluten sensitivities when they're seasoned with spices that contain gluten or served in a sauce containing wheat or other forbidden substances. The more processed the vegetables, the fancier the recipe, the more they're combined with other ingredients, the more likely something has been added for flavor-enhancement that will make it less safe, from a GF point of view. For instance, natural fries cooked in fresh oil in clean pans are safe. We love sweet potato fries, but many brands dip them into something to make them crispy—and unsafe for GF folks. So we make our own. They may not be as crispy, but they sure are safer. There are plenty of French fries and hash-browns in the frozen food section that contain only potatoes and salt. But you have to read the labels, because flavor enhancers and crispers usually have some taint of gluten in them. Baked potatoes are fine, but if they've had coatings added to make them crispy or more flavorful, these additions may contain gluten. You can easily dress up a baked potato yourself by adding a chili, broccoli, or cheese topping, or scooping the insides out to transform them into stuffed potatoes.

Do you long for crispy vegetables? You can purchase GF bread crumbs, which is what we use to make super eggplant parmesan patties or Indian pakoras. Sometimes we dip vegetables or meats in corn starch that we've seasoned and then fry them up. You can still get the tasty, crispy sensation without making someone sick.

Sauces can make vegetables more tempting and are easy to make. A cheese sauce for cauliflower or broccoli; a pasta sauce, a vinaigrette, a ranch type dressing or sauce—there's no excuse for not liking vegetables when they are so friendly for your personal adaptation and transformation.

Vegetables can also be transformed into fantastic soup. Remember the old story of stone soup? You add a little of this and a little of that, depending on what you have around, and suddenly you have a scrumptious soup. See our chapter on soup recipes if you need inspiration.

Fruits are gluten free when fresh or frozen with nothing on them. Fruits can be consumed whole, cut, or pureed into drinks, soups, and sauces. As every nutritionist will tell us, fresh fruits and vegetables are the best things we can eat.

A fresh banana, apple, grapes, or an orange will be safe. Just wash the skin and you're good to munch. But what about fruit salads? These are often in containers in the airports and convenience stores. They should be safe. Should. There's no way for you to know what type of environment they were made in and whether the cook used gloves that were never used on bread products. Unlike at a restaurant, there's no one to ask about how the fruit was prepared, because it probably came from a distant location. If the containers were marked with the GF sticker, we would feel much more comfortable about eating them. Our mantra is, "When in doubt, don't eat it."

Smoothies should be safe if blended with 100 percent juice and other fresh or frozen fruits. The question here is whether or not supplements that may contain gluten were added for protein or vitamins. Given that gluten is a protein, fruit protein smoothies aren't necessarily gluten free. If yogurt is used in the smoothie it should be safe—but some yogurts are made with syrups or substances that might contain gluten.

Fruit desserts and soups fall into the same category of concern; if they're made with whole fruits and have no gluten-containing additives to make them pretty, thicker, or tastier, then hooray! But you need to read the label or ask the cook. We find that the "coulda, shoulda, oughta" mentality isn't safe when it comes to eating foods that *could* be gluten free, *should* be, and *ought* to be if fixed right.

Be careful when buying dried fruit, because many of these products are processed in the same places where wheat products are used. While it may seem like that wouldn't be a big deal, it is if you're highly sensitive to gluten. Most dried fruits make us a little nervous. We were in an airport starving, since there was no safe restaurant food available, and we spied a little store that sold dried fruits and nuts. Aha, we thought! Dinner! Nope—the items were in large containers with no labels, so we asked the shop keeper to take a look at the bag they came in. Sure enough, they were made in a facility that also processed wheat items. Some of them even had wheat listed on the label.

Don't take a chance and put your trust in wishes—ask and find out the truth. Your body will be happy, even if the sales clerk or wait person acts annoyed. The next person who comes by and needs gluten free food will benefit because you helped inspire the clerk to consider the importance of the issue.

Meats. Chicken, fish, beef, pork and other fresh meats are fine on their own. When you purchase them, buy fresh when you can. Pieces of beef, pork, chicken or fish in their natural state look natural in their plastic or paper wraps and if they've not had anything done to alter the natural state, they're likely fine. Whether baked, fried, grilled, or cooked in natural broth, meats on their own cannot make someone with gluten sensitivities sick.

That said, like fresh vegetables, meats can become dangerous for folks with gluten intolerance when they're marinated or smothered in substances that contain gluten. Some bottled marinades are marked GF, but marinades that are pre-made in a store are seldom safe. Luckily, you can make lovely, delicious marinades at home, such as mixing lime juice and seasonings in a bowl and covering the meat for a period of time. With the high cost of unsafe store marinades, you will even save money by spending a few extra minutes creating your own product. If there's any question in your mind, don't get those pre-marinated steak tips or chicken breasts.

Know that meats that should be safe may be cross-contaminated by cooking them on surfaces that have been contaminated by wheat products, or adding seasonings that contain gluten. Cooking on the grill isn't a good idea unless you put down aluminum foil or use a clean pan on the grill. Whatever was there before lingers, unless you're a super scrubber. This means watching over where your meat is cooked, even if you're a guest at a cookout.

You should avoid processed meats, unless you're eating a gluten free Fenway Frank, because many hot dogs and cold-cuts have gluteny and mystery fillers. Cold-cuts, hot dogs, salami, sausages, etc., often have modified food starch (a code word for potential gluten in products) used to bind water into the processed meats. At our grocery, we know one brand of turkey breast is gluten free, but the rest aren't. We had to ask the clerks, and when they didn't know, they asked the managers, who found out for us. Now we all know which deli meats are safe. Products such as Boars Head pride themselves on using natural ingredients and are gluten free. Even their condiments, such as mustards, are gluten free.

Breaded chicken and fish, or meats prepared with spices that have gluten in them are not safe. Gluten free breadings are fine, but this requires buying certified GF brands or making them yourself at home. When dining out, know that most breaded meats or vegetables are not safe, so you're wise to avoid them.

Bacon is usually safe; bacon bits are usually not, so beware. Sausage is a toss-up; it all depends on where you get it, the brand, and what's in it. Sausage is one of those meats you have to know well— either ask the butcher who made it or carefully read the label. We've been surprised by the sausages, and now have a variety we know and trust—and those we don't.

We've found butchers we trust to know about gluten free ingredients and we ask them directly when we're unsure. Buying "off the rack" at the meat counters for foods that might be safe, but might not, isn't a wise idea. It may cost a little more to buy directly from a butcher who knows what's in the marinades and how the meats were processed, but there are big advantages to doing so. You're not getting sick, which is a huge benefit. You're also buying local and helping a mom-and-pop business.

Nuts. Raw nuts are always safe for people with gluten issues. Roasted nuts with a little sea salt are fine. The problem arises when nuts are doused with sweet, spicy, or crunchy coatings. The more elaborate the coating on nuts, the more risky they are. Sometimes nut coatings are safe, but usually they aren't. I've learned how to "dress them up" at home in my own kitchen with safe ingredients when I want nuts in a more elaborate state. It's easy to toast them in the microwave, the oven, or in a skillet with butter, sugar, spices, or other GF seasonings of your choice.

Another caution about nuts is whether or not they were processed on machinery that also processes wheat. Fortunately, companies are required by law to let you know this. Long ago, they didn't. Usually equipment is wiped clean between processing different batches of nuts, but wheat particles are so tiny they can lurk in gears and places that are hard to clean. While the contamination may be slight, if you're super sensitive to gluten, you could get sick. So the verdict on nuts is:

Raw: almost always gluten free

Roasted: could or could not be, so make sure to read the label

Nuts with dried fruit: likely not gluten free

Seasoned or coated nuts: probably not gluten free unless specifically noted.

Milk Products. Natural cheeses, ice cream, yogurts, butter, milk, and cream are usually safe for people with celiac disease or gluten concerns. However, lactose intolerance and gluten intolerance often occur in the same people. The biggest gluten concern with milk products are added ingredients, such as thickeners in flavored yogurt, cookies in ice cream, and flour based thickeners. Some yogurts are safe, while some are not—you need to get familiar with gluten code words and read the fine print on the ingredient list.

As always, the more processed the food, the less likely it's safe. If you make something at home you know exactly what's in it; if you buy it out, even if it's a great brand and an expensive price, don't automatically assume it's GF. For instance, an Alfredo sauce should naturally be safe because it contains butter, cream, and cheese. But what if it was thickened with a flour base? Then it won't be safe. The grocery may have "fresh" sauces that look amazing, but I don't trust them. It doesn't take long to make them and they are so much better made at home. Buying off the rack is not worth the risk.

Some forms of string cheese are super, but one day I brought home a nationally well-respected brand of smoked string cheese and discovered it was not safe. We gave it away, even though I could eat it. Chris is used to having only safe cheese in the fridge, so leaving unsafe food around increases the risk that in a non-thinking moment he might grab a piece and eat it before realizing it wasn't GF. Smoked cheeses are often a concern. Some goudas are GF and others are not. As with every other product, you need to learn about your options and choose wisely.

Nothing is more comforting than a cream soup, pudding, or thick based sauce. Any of these can easily be made gluten free milk and GF flours. You can add products like safe instant mashed potatoes for thickening soups. In fact, corn starch, tapioca, and GF flours often work better than wheat flour to make these dishes. Our mental reliance on flour as the sole way to thicken products is silly when so many other options are available.

Carbohydrates. In many cultures, meals revolve around a carbohydrate base, such as potatoes, rice, or pasta. As far as carbohydrates are concerned, rice, risotto, and potatoes are always safe. So are gluten free pastas, such as those made of corn, quiona, amaranth, millet, sorghum, potato starch, or rice. These carbs can form the basis for ethnic cuisine, including Italian food, Asian foods, Indian foods, or Mexican dishes.

While rice should always be safe, when it's pre-packaged with special seasonings, be careful. Wild rice mixtures, Cajun and Spanish rice products, and rice dishes with sauces are suspect. I make my own Spanish rice with salsa or fresh tomatoes, peppers, onions, cumin and cilantro in order to be safe. I add fresh basil, walnuts, pepper, and Parmesan cheese to my risotto instead buying the boxed version. This is easy to accomplish once you have a ready supply of different herbs and spices on hand.

In general, it's wise to think about our relationship with breads, pastas, and other carbohydrate foods. Carbs have become a source of debate and scrutiny by many in the nutrition and health communities. We're not taking a position on whether or not you should eat them (as we grew up on them and personally love them), but we've found that we've cut the amount we eat by over three-fourths and haven't missed them at all. Well, maybe a little now and then, but not enough to justify the desire.

When we first went gluten free I had no idea there was any kind of flour besides wheat. I imagine I'm not the only one who thought like that. Here's a list of flours that are gluten free:

Almond	Amaranth	Arrowroot
Buckwheat	Chestnut	Chickpeas
Coconut	Corn	Lentils
Millet	Montina	Potato
Quinoa	Rice	Sago
Sorghum	Soy	Tapioca
Teff		

Do NOT trust any of the following flours or grains: wheat, bulgur, couscous, durum, semolina, barley, rye, triticale, spelt, kamut or einkorn (Beth Isreal Deaconess Medical Center)[10].

Like me, most Americans grow up thinking wheat is the only type of flour that exists. Learning how to use different flours can open up a whole new world of cooking. For instance, homemade lemon bars may be even better when made with coconut or almond flour instead of wheat flour. Corn flour makes immensely better taco and enchilada wraps than wheat flour. Indian pakoras are especially delicious when made with garbanzo flour. Discovering the wide range of flours empowers cooks to be more creative, and the outcomes may be superior to dishes previously made with wheat flour.

The key to a healthy, gluten free diet is knowing what foods to stay away from, and how to embellish the wonderful natural foods that exist. The interesting thing about being introduced to all these other carbohydrates and grains is that it opens a door to a host of new cuisines and recipes. Instead of being deprived because you can't have wheat, you may find your diet is enhanced.

Herbs and Spices. There are plenty of ways to spice up gluten free foods. Olive oil, butter, salt, and pepper are wonderful staples. I prefer natural seasonings such as basil, cumin, rosemary, coriander, cinnamon, chili powder, or tarragon, which can make food taste wonderful. Learning how to use spices can make foods quite interesting and tasteful. In general, dried and fresh herbs should be fine. We grow

---

10   Beth Israel Deaconess. http://bit.ly/1LViWFo

many of our own, and it's possible to have an inside herb garden of herbs like basil, rosemary, thyme, and dill. This is easiest to do if you don't have a cat who may also like fresh herbs (we've found growing them their own catnip is no assurance they won't help themselves to our herbs).

When it comes to buying spices, carefully read the ingredients on the labels. Sometimes less expensive products use fillers or mixtures of different spice ingredients that may contain gluten. Here is a brief run-down on spice GF safety: http://dld.bz/d6are

Durkee sells 92 different spices processed on dedicated lines that aren't used for gluten-containing items. Make sure to read ingredients on their blends; while most spice blends are safe, if it says "modified food starch" it's probably corn, but check to make sure. McCormick states that it tries to process products on separate lines and will declare if it uses wheat, barley, rye or oats in its ingredients list.

Frontier Co-op spices have eliminated all known gluten from their facility. Magic Seasonings says its blends are considered GF at 20 parts per million except for Breading Magic and Gumbo Gravy Magic. I'll be honest—if I'm not totally sure the spices are safe, I don't use them. Most of the time, well-cooked food is delicious without them.

Commonly Consumed Food Products

Almost everyone has favorite foods they wouldn't want to live without. Here is a short list of commonly foods you may wonder about.

Alcohol

Perhaps you like to have a glass of wine, a bottle of beer, or a mixed drink now and then. However, many alcohol drinks aren't safe for people with gluten issues. Whiskey, rum, and gin are often safe, depending on the brand. Products in the beer family are made with malt, wheat, or barley, and therefore are not safe for anyone with gluten intolerance. However gluten free beers are available for those people who've just gotta have it. The list of safe alcoholic beverages includes:

- Armagnac, which is made from grapes, is safe.
- Against the Grain, World Top Brewery (United Kingdom)
- Bards Tale Dragons Gold, Bard's Tale Beer Company (USA)
- BeerUp Glutenfrei, Grieskirchen (Austria)
- Birra 76 Bi-Aglut, Heineken Italy (Italy)
- Blonde (also Ginger and Apple Beers), Billabong Brewing (Australia)
- Daura, Estrella Damm (Spain)
- G-Free, St. Peter's Brewery (United Kingdom)
- Green's Endeavour Dubble, Green's (United Kingdom)
- Koff I, Sinebrychoff (Finland)
- Lammsbräu, Neumarkter (Germany)
- Messagère, Les bières de la Nouvelle-France (Canada)
- Mongozo's exotic flavorded pilsners (The Netherlands)
- New Grist, Lakefront Brewery (USA)
- Nodogoshi, Kirin (Japan)
- O'Brien Brown Ale, O'Brien Brewery (Australia)
- Passover Honey Beer, Ramapo Valley (USA)
- RedBridge, Anheuser-Busch (USA)
- Residenz Bio-Reis-Gold Dunkel, Liebharts (Germany)
- Schnitzer Bräu (Germany)
- Sorghum Molasses Brown, Outer Banks (USA)
- Toleration, Hambleton (United Kingdom)
- Tread Lightly Ale and 3R Raspberry Ale, New Planet (USA)
- Tumma Kukko, Laitilan (Finland)
- Bourbon, especially from *Makers Mark*, tends to be safe.
- Brandy in general is safe.
- Champagne, made from grapes, may be safe.
- Cider, fermented from apples or other fruits, may be safe. For a list of GF brands, see http://bit.ly/1ae2Ta7

- Cognac is made from grapes so it is usually safe.
- Gin
- Grappa
- Kahlua
- Kirschwasser (cherry liqueur)
- Martini: *Club Extra Dry Martini* (corn & grape) or *Club Vodka Martini* (corn & grape).
- Mead wine tends to be safe, as it is distilled from honey.
- Mistico, especially *Jose Cuervo Mistico* (agave and cane).
- Mixes and cooking alcohol:
  - *Club Tom Collins* (corn).
  - *Diamond Jims Bloody Mary Mystery.*
  - *Holland House* - all EXCEPT Teriyaki Marinade and Smooth & Spicy Bloody Mary Mixes.
  - *Mr. & Mrs. T* - all Except Bloody Mary Mix.
  - *Spice Islands* - Cooking Wines - Burgundy, Sherry and White.
  - Margarita Mix tends to be safe, especially those made by *Jose Cuervo or Mr. & Mrs. T.*
- Ouzo - made from grapes and anise.
- Rum
- Sake is fermented with rice and Koji enzymes. The Koji enzymes are grown on Miso, which is usually made with barley. The two-product separation from barley and the manufacturing process should make it safe for people with Celiac.
- Scotch whiskey
- Sherry
- Sparkling wine
- Tequila
- Vermouth - distilled from grapes.
- Vodka
- Wine - all wines, including port wines and sherry, are safe.

Because so many types of alcohol may have additives or be mixed with other ingredients, Chris finds alcohol products aren't worth the risk. Drinking is always a matter of personal preference.

Pre-made breads

Bread may be regarded as the staff of life, but wheat bread can make people with celiac disease feel like they're going to die. I grew up making wheat bread like my mom and her mother before her, and must say with pride that mine was even better than theirs. However, when it comes to making homemade gluten free bread, what I make isn't even close in quality. My loaves are heavy, I find it doesn't rise right, and even after experimenting with a variety of different products, I haven't found one that meets my standards. I recently discussed this with the baker at Blackberry Bakery in Londonderry, NH who agrees that making high-quality gluten free bread is a challenge.

As long as we expect gluten free bread to be exactly like wheat bread, we're probably in for disappointment. But if we change our expectations and cooking styles, then we may find the breads are more satisfying. I find it easier to buy unsliced GF bread, but I'm betting it's only a matter of time before a superior sliced bread product becomes widely available.

Fortunately, many products are now available to help you create your own GF bread. The King Arthur Flour Company, which is famous for empowering bakers to make outstanding products for generations, has created a dedicated line of GF products. In my opinion, theirs are the best on the market, although their breads still aren't as good as their gluten products.

In the frozen bread category, Udi and Against The Grain companies sell delicious frozen GF food products, including bagels, pizza crusts, and breads. The Bob's Red Mill brand, 123 Gluten free, Glutino, and other gluten free brands produce fine products that enable people with celiac disorders to enjoy bread and bread products.

Cakes and cookies

While making home-made bread can be challenging, creating delectable gluten free cakes, muffins, brownies, and cookies is easy. Many amazing products are on the market, and more surface all the time. The Betty Crocker and King Arthur brownie and cookie mixes are delicious. I find it easier to create good cakes by adding special ingredients such as carrot shreads, chocolate chips, poppy seeds with almond extract, or peanut butter to make products that are similar to the baked goods we used to make with wheat flour. I use GF crushed pecan or shortbread cookies as a crust for lemon bars and cheesecakes, and these are more than satisfactory.

The biggest trick for baking cakes and cookies is the Goldilocks strategy—cooking them too short a time makes for soggy middles, while baking too long makes them rock hard. The issue is finding that "just right" cooking time—but that issue is the same for wheat-based bakers too. While we may buy GF Oreo type cookies or fancy bakery birthday cakes, we whip up most other types of baked desserts in our own kitchen and find them easy and delicious, especially when served right out of the oven.

Candy

Most people have a sweet tooth, and depriving ourselves of sweets can make us cranky and miserable on a GF diet. Here is an online list of candies that are thought to be safe: http://bit.ly/19w4bfI

The following list will help you make a safe decision about what candy to buy:

AIRHEADS – In general, Airheads candy does not contain peanuts, tree nuts, pine nuts, sesame, eggs or dairy; however, since it would not be typical for these items to be found in the products, they perform no specific test for them. Airheads Bars are free of peanuts, tree nuts, egg, milk, wheat/gluten but are manufactured in a facility that processes wheat flour. Airheads Xtremes Belts contain wheat flour and wheat starch.

AMERICAN LICORICE CO. – Products such as Sour Punch Twists, Bites, Red, Black or Fruit Vines do contain gluten and wheat, but do not contain peanuts, tree nuts or sesame and peanut oil. In general, stay away from licorice. We have a seen gluten free black licorice before, but it's hard to find. Red is seldom safe for people who need to stay away from gluten.

ANGIE'S ARTISAN TREATS – Kettle Corn does not contain any of the top eight allergens and is certified gluten free.

ANNABELLE'S – Their only guaranteed gluten free candy is the 2 oz. Big Hunk. For all other candies, including the mini Big Hunks, there is the possibility of contamination. While no flour is used specifically for the Big Hunk minis, flour is used on the belts for the manufacture of the Look bars. Products such as Abba Zabba, Rocky Road, and U-No may not contain gluten, but are possibly contaminated because wheat is used in their facility.

BAZOOKA – Their gum, Ring Pops, Push Pops, and Baby Bottle Pops do not contain any of the top eight allergens, and contain no wheat, gluten, or nut products. Hooray for Bazooka Joe!

CE DE CANDY – Makers of Smarties. None of their products contain any of the top eight allergens and are gluten and nut free.

CRACKER JACK – Cracker Jack is gluten free, unlike some caramel-type corn products.

FARLEY'S AND SATHERS – Makers of a variety of familiar candies, they do not use any gluten, wheat, or nut products in their candy, but they cannot certify that they are entirely safe because they can't be sure about wheat or nut contamination in the manufacturing area. Their no-gluten products include Brach's Candy Corn, Brach's Mellowcreme Pumpkins and Indian Corn, Flooders, Jujyfruits, Jujubes, Red Raspberry Dollars, Red Hot Dollars Wild Cherry, Heide Gummi Bears, Now and Later, Rain-Blo Pops, Super Bubble, or Tarolli Gummi Bears, and Trolli Sour Brite (Frite) Crawlers.

FERRARA PAN – They make Lemonhead, Red Hots, Apple/Grape/Cherry head, All Jujus, All Jelly Beans, Sour Jacks, Cherry

Sours, Boston Baked Beans, Atomic Fireballs, Gum Drops and Jawbreakers (Jawbusters) candies. They do not use wheat or gluten in their products. Nut or soy products may be manufactured in their facility, but Ferrara Pan's Allergen Policy requires a thorough, monitored cleaning of the common use lines when switching from allergen-containing products to non-allergen-containing products, and requires multi-departmental inspections as well as stringent verification procedures.

FLIX – Manufacturer of Disney Lollipop Rings. They use no wheat/gluten, peanuts, tree nuts, egg, milk, soy, or ingredients that contain the top eight allergens.

FRANKFORD CANDY & CHOCOLATE COMPANY – Their SpongeBob Gummy Krabby Patties do not contain wheat or nuts, but are manufactured in China in a facility that processes wheat and nuts. Their Marvel Super Hero candy does not contain any wheat or allergens.

GALERIE – Star Wars Lollipops contain no wheat/gluten, peanuts, tree nuts, egg, or milk products.

GOETZE'S – They make Carmel Cream and Cow Tales which DO contain wheat/gluten.

HARIBO – Most Haribo products, such as Gold Bears, are gluten free. The following Haribo products are NOT gluten free: Black Licorice Wheels, Red Licorice Wheels, Sour S'ghetti, Fruity Pasta, Brixx, Konfekt and Pontefract Cakes.

HERR'S – Their Chocolate Mini Pretzels DO contain wheat and gluten.

HERSHEY – Their following products are gluten free, including: Hershey Kisses, Hershey Bars, Baby Ruth, Bliss candies, Good & Fruity, Heath Minis, Jolly Rancher candies, Milk Duds, Mr. Goodbar, Pay Day, Reese's Peanut Butter products, Rolo, and York Peppermint Patties. Their following products MAY contain gluten: Almond Joy, Mounds, Cookies 'n' Cream products, Good & Plenty,

Take 5, Twizzlers, and Whoppers. Hershey has strict procedures in place to prevent crossover of allergens into other products.

IMPACT CONFECTIONS – Gluten free products include: Warheads, Grubs, Juniors, QBZ, Sour Spray, Spray with Lollipop, Alien Pop, Baseball Pop, Basketball Pop, Boo Pop, Carousel Pop, ColorBlaster Pop, Football Pop, Happy Heart Pop, Hoppin' Pop, Lickin' Lips Pop, Lolliday Pop, Lollinotes, Pop-A-Bear, Soccer Pop, Alien Glow Pop, Buggin' Glow Pop, Burstin Bits, Ghostly Glow Pop, Hot Tamales Spray, Ice Cream Dipper (Blue Raspberry, Strawberry), Mike and Ike Spray, Sidewalk Chalk, Sno-Cone, Soda Pop, Twist and Glow, Twist and Glow Heart, Twist and Glow Pumpkin, Gummy Brush Paint Shop, Lollipop Paint Shop, Bubble Gum Burstin' Bits. Their following products do contain gluten: Ice Cream Dipper (Cherry Cream, Vanilla Cream).

JELLY BELLY – Jelly Belly Jelly Beans are gluten free and contain none of top the eight allergens.

JUST BORN – Gluten free products include Hot Tamales, Mike and Ike, Peanut Chews Original and Milk Chocolate, Peeps.

KELLOGG'S – Their traditional Rice Krispies contain gluten, but they have developed a gluten free product line, so be aware which ones you select.

KRAFT FOODS (including CADBURY ADAMS) – Their following candies are gluten free: Jet Puffed Marshmallows, Swedish Fish, and Sour Patch products. It has been a long standing policy for all Kraft and Nabisco products to list ingredients that contain gluten on the ingredient statement.

MARS – The following products are gluten free: 3 Musketeers and 3 Musketeers Mint, Dove chocolates, M & Ms (except for M & Ms Pretzels), Milky Way Dark/Midnight Bars, Milky Way Simply Caramel and Snickers. The following products do contain gluten: Milky Way Bar, Twix.

MELSTER – The following products are gluten free: Peanut Butter Kisses.

NECCO – The following candies are gluten free: Mary Janes, Necco Wafers, Mary Jane Peanut Butter Kisses, Sweethearts Conversation Hearts (Valentines only), Canada Mint & Wintergreen Lozenges, Haviland Thin Mints and Candy Stix. In addition, Clark Bars, Skybars, Haviland Peppermint & Wintergreen Patties, Necco Candy Eggs (Easter), Talking Pumpkins (Halloween), Squirrel Nut Caramels and Squirrel Nut Zippers, Banana Split and Mint Julep Chews, Ultramints are also gluten free.

NESTLE – The following items are gluten free: Baby Ruth, Bit-O-Honey, Butterfinger, Raisinets. The following items DO contain gluten: 100 Grand, Butterfinger Crisp, Butterfinger Snackerz, Crunch, Kit Kats.

OAK LEAF – Sixlets Candy Coated Chocolate Flavored Candy and Bubble Gum are gluten free.

PEZ – Pez products are gluten free, with no chance of cross contamination since it is the only product made in their facility.

R.M. PALMER COMPANY – Their Palmer Tricky Treats (Googly Eyes, Boneheads, Pumpkin Discs), Peppermint Patties, and Peanut Butter Creepy Peepers are gluten free, but made on equipment the also processes wheat and nuts. The following products are NOT gluten free: Double Crisp Creepy Crawlies.

RIVIERA – Their Spooky Candy Rings are gluten free. These candies are NOT gluten free: Gummy Body Parts (fingers, noses), Creepy Meals, and Halloween Gummies (Spiders, Pumpkins, Ghosts, Witches).

RUSSELL STOVER – Their products tend to be gluten free, with the exception of those containing cookies, such as S'mores and Cookies and Creams. Items like Marshmallow Pumpkin, Orange Marshmallow Pumpkin, Marshmallow Football, and Coconut Cream Pumpkins are gluten free.

SPANGLER – hese products are gluten free: Dum Dums, Chewy Pops, Saf-T-Pops, Circus Peanuts, Candy Canes, Chewy Canes, Shrek Ogreheads.

STORCK – Riesen products contain wheat/gluten and are not safe for people who need gluten free foods.

TOOTSIE – The following candies are gluten free: Andes Crème de Menthe, Caramel Apple Pops, Charleston Chews, Charms Blow Pops, Dots, Dubble Bubble Bubble Gum, Tear Jerker Sour Bubble Gum, Charms Blow Pop Bubble Gum, Dubble Bubble Twist, Cry Baby Sour Gumballs, Gumballs, Painterz, Junior Mints, Junior Caramels, Tootsie Pops, Tootsie Rolls, Sugar Babies, Sugar Mamas, and Sugar Daddy.

WELCH'S – Their Fruit Snacks are gluten free.

WRIGLEY – Their following items are gluten free: Altoids (except for Altoids Smalls Peppermint), CremeSavers, Hubba Bubba Gum, Life Savers, Life Savers Gummies, Skittles, and Starburst. The following items are NOT gluten free: Hubba Bubba Gummy Tape and Altoids Smalls Peppermint.

WONKA – These candies are wheat/gluten free: Bottlecaps, Everlasting Glbstopers, Fun Dip, Pixy Stix, Runts, Laffy Taffy (not stretchy), and Giant Chewy Nerds. Sweetarts and Nerds do not contain gluten but are made in a facility that also processes wheat, so cross contamination is possible. These contain gluten: Kazoozles, Sweetarts Gummy Bugs.

ANNIE'S – Their Organic Bunny Fruit Snacks (Flavors: Tropical Treat, Berry Patch, Sunny Citrus, Summer Strawberry) are gluten free.

CRISPY CAT – These items are gluten free: Mint Coconut Candy Bar, Toasted Almond Candy Bar, and Chocolate Sundae Candy Bar.

SURF SWEETS – Gummy Worms, Gummy Swirls, Gummy Bears, Fruity Bears, Jelly Beans, Sour Worms, and Sour Berry Bears are gluten free.

In general, we always have candy around and never feel deprived. Giving up foods you love isn't healthy if it makes you feel like you're in jail.

Condiments

Did you know that Heinz ketchup is safe for people with celiac disease, but many other ketchup brands are not? From the consumer's point of view, knowing Heinz is safe means that a bottle marked Heinz ought to be okay—right? Sometimes in restaurants Heinz ketchup bottles are filled each night, but the restaurant may pour into them from cans of less expensive ketchup. This is where the issue of transparency arises again. Restaurants shouldn't put out products with incorrect labels. Better to pour the cheap ketchup into a red plastic squirt bottle that clearly states "generic" than to intentionally mislead customers who depend upon accurate labeling.

Likewise, mustard can be a questionable condiment, but French's Mustard, like Boars Head condiments, are safe. Other condiments, dressings, or sauce brands that are typically safe for gluten sensitive people include Franks Original Red-Hot, Organicville, Maple Grove Farms, Seeds of Change, San-J, and Premier Japan.

With hundreds of condiments, dressings, sauces, and marinades on the market, it's impossible to list them all; look on the label or go to the product's web site. If a product has the GF logo on it, or states it is gluten free, buy it; otherwise, choose a product you know is safe, or improvise by making your own.

Dressings and dips

The standard rule holds true: If you make salad dressings or dips yourself, you know they're fresh and safe for gluten free eaters, but you buy them at your own risk unless they're specifically marked gluten free. Never forget to read the label. Some dressings aren't marked gluten free, but they are. The company probably just hasn't gone through the certification process.

I love my own salad dressings more than any products from the grocery. My homemade dressings are delicious, natural, easy to make, and inexpensive because I use olive oil, vinegars, spices, and produce I have on hand. Check out our recipe chapter for how we make our dressings. I bet you'll love them!

As for dips, we tend not to buy them because they're often thickened or "tastied up" with products containing gluten. The exception is hummus, which is almost always GF. Dips made at home without glutened substances are fresh and wonderful. Certain dip mixes are gluten free, but—have you gotten the message yet?—you need to look around, read the ingredients, and stick with the ones that are safe.

Gravies and sauces

Sauces can make a meal fantastic, or boring. We initially missed eating sauces because most of them weren't gluten free. You'll find it's easy to whip up tasty sauces in your own kitchen. Homemade Alfredo and cream sauces are easy to make and can be thickened with corn starch or a variety of non-wheat flours. In general, when we eat out we avoid sauces, dips, and dressings entirely. Unless we have a direct conversation with the chef or manager who assures us he sauces are made "from scratch" and all ingredients are known to be gluten free, we don't take a chance. Pre-bottled sauces that are certified gluten free are fine, but most commercial sauces leave consumers not knowing for sure. Stubbs brands barbeque sauces are gluten free and delicious.

Soy sauce is a commonly used staple in Asian foods that usually contains wheat. We avoid going out for Chinese food most of the time unless we're confident the restaurant uses gluten free soy sauce. Many brands exist; just remember to check for gluten free on the label. Since the gluten free soy sauces are just as good as regular soy sauces, it makes sense to purchase gluten free soy sauce for all cooking. This eliminates any possibility of contamination.

We thought if soy sauce was generally unsafe, soy itself might be a problem. So we stayed away from it for years. But according to experts at the Healthy Villi, soy is safe. This means that plain tofu, soy flour, and ingredients made from soy should be fine. Good to know!

In many ways, gravy and sauces are similar. Gravy can be a lovely addition to meals. Look for gluten free products—or better yet, make your own from broth and corn starch. We'll show you the recipes later in this book. But sometimes we're in a hurry and using something pre-made may be easier. Be careful. Gravies that are the "just add water" packet type and those that come in open-and-serve jars often contain wheat based thickeners. White sauces are a staple in cooking, and they can easily be made with butter mixed with non-wheat flours, such as the all-purpose gluten free flour by King Arthur. Then add milk, salt, and pepper until the gravy is smooth and delicious.

Drinks

Obviously, water is safe, and so are 100 percent juices. Milk, for those who aren't lactose intolerant, is fine. The more complicated the drinks, the more need for awareness of their ingredients. Coffee is usually acceptable, but be wary of exotic flavorings. Teas should also be fine, but some teas are flavored with gluten containing ingredients. Certain brands of green tea may contain barley. Read the box, or go to sites like Celiac.com where you can find a list of safe products.

Soft drinks made with sugar or corn syrup may be fine, but sometimes sodas contain flavor enhancers that render them unsafe. For instance, one day I bought a Jones New York blue-raspberry soda and brought it home, only to find Chris writhing in distress after drinking it. Who knew someone would add glutened products to a soft drink? As a general rule, the purer and simpler a drink, the greater the chance it is safe; the more exotic it is, the more you need to check the ingredients. See http://dld.bz/d6Euu for a list of GF sodas.

Eggs

If you crack the egg yourself, it doesn't contain gluten. Fake eggs or egg whites in pourable containers are usually safe, but always read the ingredients of any new product to know for sure. When dining out, make sure the eggs aren't embellished with fillers to make them fluffy. Eggs on their own are gluten free, so they should be safe to eat in any form.

Fast foods

As a general rule, most fast foods are not gluten free, but if you shop carefully most fast food restaurants have something on the menu that's safe. It depends entirely on where you go. Several websites list fast food chains and gluten information, including: http://dld.bz/dzeJq and http://dld.bz/dzeJu.

In general, fries are usually not safe when cooked in the same oil as chicken tenders. Curly fries have a special salt mixture that may contain gluten. Many of the meats aren't 100 percent meat and contain gluten fillers. Some of the chickens and meats are made of slurry, which has almost no meat and is mostly filler. The batters and coatings commonly used on fast foods may make them crispy and delicious, but they aren't gluten free. Even salads and yogurt items may not be safe, but they could be. You'll need to do your homework and find out. Ice cream is often the most common gluten free product at a fast food restaurant. Wendy's chili or baked potatoes are gluten free.

Do fast food restaurants have gluten free options? Yes. But the lack of diversity in most fast food joints is amazing.

As naturopathic docto Duffy McKay pointed out, the best fast food ever is an apple or piece of string cheese. Those items are safe. A little planning and packing ahead, or stopping in a grocery instead of the restaurant, can make a world of difference when you need to grab something quick to eat.

Ice cream

A variety of wonderful ice creams are available, and so long as they don't contain thickeners or gluten items like crunchy cookies or cookie dough, they should be fine. Bryers and Edy's Ice Creams, Talenti, and Haagen Dazs are sensitive to gluten issues. Dove ice cream chocolate covered bars are also safe, as are Reese's peanut butter ice creams. Klondike bars and Magnum Bars (unless cookie covered) tend to be safe, as are York Peppermint Pattie ice creams and Reeses Peanut Butter Cup ice cream. Gelatos and sorbets are usually safe as well. Ben and Jerry's don't label their ice creams gluten free, but they are clear about the ingredients. If you can read and decipher what's gluten from what isn't, you should be able to figure out which of their ice creams are safe. Check the contents to make sure they don't contain contaminants, like pretzel, cookie, or brownie pieces. In general, simple ice creams are usually safe.

Soup

Canned soups may not be gluten free. Homemade soups are safe, if you make them that way. Whether a tomato base, chicken broth, chili, or cream based soups, these can be made easily in your own kitchen with wholesome ingredients and no fear of gluten contamination. While some canned soups may be gluten free, they don't compare in quality with homemade soup. See the recipe chapter for ideas.

If you must eat canned soup, some brands are better than other for gluten free options. This web page contains a list of gluten free soups: http://dld.bz/dzeJU. Twenty of Amy's 29 soups are gluten free; many Progresso soups are safe, and so are the Wolfgang Puck soups that are labeled gluten free. Unfortunately, Campbell Soup Company does not make the gluten free list.

Vinegar

Vinegar is a curious product, with considerable debate on what is safe. Ideally, distilled vinegar should gluten free, which means any product (like pickles) made with it should be gluten free as well. White vinegar was a product under debate for its gluten free safety, but according to the Healthy Villi experts, all vinegar is now considered safe with the exception of malt vinegar. Apple cider vinegar is universally regarded as safe. Balsamic vinegar is usually thought to be safe as well. When in doubt, stick with cider vinegar products in order to ensure no inadvertent contamination.

Surprising Items to Check for Gluten

We assumed gluten was only found in food until Chris used a shampoo that made his body break out in a horrible rash. The dermatitis was almost like a burn on his head, ears, neck, and where the soap ran down his chest and back. Another time he got sick by taking a vitamin pill we only later learned was not gluten free. People with gluten sensitivity need to know that gluten may also be present in items we'd never suspect, including beverages, vitamins, lipstick, lip balm, dental products, lotion, and shampoo. You may find it annoying to check the ingredients in these products, but honestly, which is more annoying—taking three minutes to look up ingredients or spending the next 24 hours feeling sick?

Did you know that some medicines contain gluten? The website www.glutenfreedrugs.com may be helpful for you to if the medications you take are gluten free. Compounding pharmacists can mix your medicines so they contain only safe ingredients for you. Check out www.iacprx.org.

Medicines that are supposed to make you feel better can make you sick if they include gluten, Chris has developed a relationship with a local pharmacist who mixes his medication so it won't contain gluten products.

Ingredients: Safe or Not?

Besides regular food items, most cooks use special ingredients to make their foods taste better. Some nutritionists warn that if an ingredient can't be easily pronounced or is longer than three syllables, a cook or consumer should be wary. These ingredients are probably not natural, which makes them troublesome for people with food allergies.

Here is a list of ingredients, by alphabetical order, that are usually safe for people with gluten intolerance. Scott Adams, at Celiac.com, was the source for most of this list.

Safe ingredients

Acacia Gum	Agar	Agave
Albumen	Alfalfa	Algae
Algin	Almond Nut	Apple Cider Vinegar
Arabic Gum	Arrowroot	Artichokes
Balsamic Vinegar	Beans	BHA, BHT
Bicarbonate of Soda	Blue Cheese	Brown Sugar
Butter (ck additives)	Cane Sugar	Canola Oil
Channa (Chickpea)	Carob	Cheeses (ck ingred)
Chestnuts	Chickpea	Cocoa
Coconut	Corn Masa Flour	Corn Meal and Flour
Corn Starch	Corn Sugar	Corn Syrup
Corn Vinegar	Cream of Tartar	Dal (Lentils)
Dates	Eggs	Fish (fresh)
Fruit (incl. dried)	Garbanzo Beans	Gelatin
Grits, Corn	Herbs	Hominy
Honey	Horseradish (Pure)	Jowar (Sorghum)
Kudzu	Lecithin	Lemon Grass
Lentils	Licorice	Maize
Masa	Masa Harina	Meat (fresh)
Milk	Oils and Fats	Peas
Peanuts	Peppers	Polenta
Potatoes	Potato Flour	Quinoa
Rice	Soy	Soybean
Spices (pure)	Tapioca	Tea
Tofu (Soy Curd)	Whey	

Unsafe Ingredients: Avoid these foods if you have celiac disease or gluten sensitivity

Atta Flour	Barley	Bleached Flour
Bran	Brewer's Yeast	Brown Flour
Bulgur Wheat/Nuts	Cereal Binding	Chilton
Couscous	Dinkle (Spelt)	Durum wheat (Triticum durum)

Edible Starch

Einkorn (Triticum monococcum)

Emmer (Triticum dicoccon)

Enriched Bleached Wheat Flour

Farina

Farro

Filler

Fu (dried wheat gluten)

Germ

Graham Flour

Granary Flour

Groats

Hard Wheat

Heeng

Hing

Kamut

Kecap Manis

Kluski Pasta

Maida (Indian wheat flour)

Malt

Macha Wheat (Triticum aestivum)

Matzo

Meringue

Meripro

Mir

Nishasta

Oriental Wheat (Triticum turanicum)

Orzo Pasta

Pasta

Pearl Barley

Persian Wheat (Triticum carthlicum)

Perungayam

Poulard Wheat (Triticum turgidum)

Polish Wheat (Triticum polonicum)

Rice Malt

Roux

Rusk

Rye

Seitan

Semolina

Shot Wheat (Triticum aestivum)

Spelt (Triticum spelta)

Sprouted Wheat or Barley

Stearyldimonium-hydroxypropyl Hydrolyzed Wheat Protein

Tabbouleh /Tabouli

Teriyaki Sauce

Timopheevi Wheat (Triticum timopheevii)

Triticale X triticosecale

Triticum Vulgare l

Udon

Unbleached Flour

Vavilovi Wheat (Triticum aestivum)

Vital Wheat Gluten

Wheat, Abyssinian Hard triticum durum

Wheat

Wheat Bran Extract

Wheat, Bulgur

Wheat Durum Triticum

Wheat Germ Extract, glycerides, oil

Wheat Grass

Wheat Nuts

Wheat Protein

Whole-meal Flour

Wild Einkorn (Triticum boeotictim)

Wild Emmer (Triticum dicoccoides)

Questionable ingredients

Many ingredients are suspicious and may contain gluten—or not. While some of the following ingredients may be safe for people with gluten intolerance, it's best to stay away from them unless one knows for sure they're safe.

Artificial Color	Baking powder	Clarifying Agents
Dextrins	Dry Roasted Nuts	Emulsifiers
Fat Replacer	Flavoring	Food Starch
Glucose Syrup	Hydrolyzed Protein	Hydroxypropylated Starch
Maltose	Miso	Mixed Tocopherols
Modified Food Starch	Natural Flavoring	Natural Juices
Non-dairy Creamer	Protein Hydrolysates	Seafood Analogs
Seasonings	Sirimi	Liquid Smoke Flavoring
Soba Noodles	Soy Sauce	Stabilizers
Starch	Suet	Tocopherols
Vegetable broth, protein, starch	Vitamins	Wheat Starch

Food Warnings

Fortunately for all of us, the government is encouraging food producers to be more transparent about what's in their products. In August 2013, the FDA ruled that in order to label an item gluten free, it must be tested to prove the amount of contaminant is under 20 parts per million (ppm). In order to better understand what 20 ppm is, Healthy Villi gives this example: Take a 1 ounce slice of bread and cut it into 7,030 pieces. Each of those tiny pieces equals 20 ppm.

The law indicates that wheat or gluten items must be listed on food labels. This is a leap forward from the "modified food starch" issue. Until this law went into effect, we had no way of knowing what the modified food starch was made from. Now it typically means corn, but if gluten is used, the labels have to say so. The names of food allergens must also appear. So when you read the label, an ingredient may have parentheses behind it with the name of the ingredient, such as "lecithin (soy)," "flour (wheat)," or "whey (milk)." Labels may also include a statement like "Contains wheat and soy," or "Made in a facility that also processes wheat."

Gluten free products and companies

Here is a partial list of gluten free websites and product distributors that may be of interest to cooks and consumers. Most of us get our favorite products from many different companies, so trial and error is the most realistic recommendation we can make. We could tell you our favorites, but that might dissuade you from trying others you would enjoy more. New vendors and products emerge all the time, so regard the list as only a suggestion and always be adventurous to try to new products when you learn of them. Some are absolutely fantastic and enjoyed by everyone, irrespective of dietary needs.

123 Gluten free – http://www.123glutenfree.com/: Mixes for breads, pancakes and other gluten free products.

Against The Grain - http://againstthegraingourmet.com/: Breads, pizza

Allergy Free Foods – http://allergyfreefoods.elsstore.com/: Chicken tenders

Ashera's Gluten free Foods – http://www.asherahsgourmet.com/: Vegan burgers, etc

Authentic Foods – http://authenticfoods.com/: Flours and mixes for baking, falafel mix

Bell and Evans – http://www.bellandevans.com/: Gluten free Chicken that is awesome!

Better Batter – http://betterbatter.org/: Flour products and mixes for baking

Bob's Red Mill – http://www.bobsredmill.com/: Mixes, flours, grains, etc.

Breads From Anna – www.breadsfromanna.com: Bread and other flour type mixes

Cause You're Special – http://www.causeyourespecial.com/: Baked goods mixes.

Chebe – http://www.chebe.com/: Cheese bread, cinnamon roll,

focaccia, and other mixes

Dr. Schar Gluten free Foods – http://www.schar.com: Breads, crackers, pizza crust, cookies, coatings, etc.

Emmy's Organics – http://emmysorganics.com/: Granola, cookies, cakes, pie mix, chocolate sauce, etc.

Enjoy Life – http://www.enjoylifefoods.com/: Cookies, cereals, snack bars, trail mix, etc.

Foods Alive – http://www.foodsalive.com/: Flax crackers, hemp based foods, etc.

Gluten freeda – http://www.glutenfreeda.com: Oats, cereals, wraps, desserts, burritos, cheesecake, etc.

Glutino – http://www.glutino.com/: Frozen meals, crackers, cookies, breads, mixes, etc.

Go Macro – http://www.gomacro.com/: Snack bars and treats

The Grainless Baker - http://www.thegrainlessbaker.com/: Bread, pasta, muffins, pastries, etc.

Kay's Naturals – http://www.kaysnaturals.com/: Cereal, cookies, pretzels, etc.

King Arthur – http://www.kingarthurflour.com/glutenfree/: Flours and gluten free baking mixes of all sorts.

Mrs. Crimbles – http://www.mrscrimbles.com/: Gourmet cookies, crackers, and mixes

Mrs. Mays – http://www.mrsmays.com/: Trio bars, crunches, chips, sesame strips, etc.

Natural Nectar – http://www.natural-nectar.com/: Crackers, cookies, lady fingers, chocolate spreads, etc.

Ogran – http://www.orgran.com/: Pasta, crackers, cookies, mixes

Perdue – http://www.perdue.com/simplysmartglutenfree/: Chicken tenders

RP's Pasta Company – http://www.rpspasta.com/gluten free-pasta/: Homemade fusilli and linguini

Shabati – http://www.shabtai-gourmet.com/: Specializes in gourmet gluten free desserts

Shiloh Farms – http://www.shilohfarms.com/: Flours and mixes

Simple Squares – http://www.simplesquares.com: Snack bars

Udi's – http://udisglutenfree.com/: Bread, bagels, pizza crust, granola, etc.

From a shopper's point of view, your options needn't be limited by where you live. Geography once dictated shopping options, but with online stores, shopping is easy and products can be delivered directly to your door. For example, Gluten free Mall (www.Glutenfreemall .com) offers online shopping for major gluten free products. With fabulous websites like this, there's no excuse for not having delicious gluten free products.

A host of different books help shoppers locate gluten free foods. *Cecelia's Marketplace Gluten free Grocery Shopping Guide* is updated annually (http://www.ceceliasmarketplace.com/gluten free-guide/) Triumph Dining offers *The Essential Gluten Free Grocery Guide* and *The Essential Gluten Free Restaurant Guide* (http://www.triumphdining.com/).

Summary

Eating gluten free is easy if you follow a natural diet devoid of wheat products. This is the "defeat the wheat" strategy. Vegetables, fruits, meats, milk products, rice, corn, and even many name-brand candies are absolutely safe. The problem comes when we move away from simple foods, because many processed and pre-packaged foods are still a concern for people who need to eat gluten free. Transforming your buying habits to move away from processed and contaminated food to foods that are safe for everyone is not only easy, it's also healthier for you and your family.

We've added a host of GF staples to our diet—things we keep on hand or buy on a regular basis. Having a well-stocked pantry makes it easy to whip up delicious foods without having to think twice. Running to the store every time you want to cook gluten free can be annoying indeed. So don't plan to be annoyed—plan to be organized and create easy, happy culinary outcomes.

Most cooks realize they have problems making certain dishes and it is easier to buy these products. For instance, the Blackberry Bakery in Londonderrry, NH makes exquisite gluten free cakes that are just as beautiful and tasty as regular wheat-based cakes. I feel as though my cheesecakes and brownies are better than any I can buy anywhere, but their GF macaroons and cakes are superior to mine. We love their almond horns so much that I learned to make them and I'm willing to put mine against theirs now. Udi's GF bagels are wonderful, far better than I could make. We keep Rosemary French Bread baguettes from Against the Grain stashed in the freezer to pull out for a quick but to-die-for bruschetta by merely tossing on a little olive oil, fresh basil, tomatoes, and Italian cheese. My pizzas are pretty fine, but in a hurry, the frozen Against The Grain pesto pizza is marvelous. I toss it into the oven and we can all do a last-minute pizza dinner.

The bottom line is, we cook amazingly delicious meals every day, and they just happen to be gluten free. When we first started being GF, we didn't know what we were doing. We spent too much money on products that were not so tasty. Now we shop and cook in a way that's easy, convenient, and so good. You can do the same.

Chapter 3

*What Happens In the Kitchen
Doesn't Stay in the Kitchen*

YOUR KITCHEN MAY BE a cook's paradise, but now you need to set everything up for gluten free food. I grew up in the kitchen, with wheat products the center around which the rest of the menu revolved. Every day I watched my mother whip up dumplings, homemade noodles, pot pies, cake, cookies, fruit pies, and dinner rolls. Her canister of flour lived on the cabinet where all foods were prepared. I naturally assumed the wheat flour canister should be on my counter also—which meant every time I opened it particles wafted into the air and landed who knows where.

Transforming my kitchen into a gluten free zone took a little bit of adjustment, mentally and physically. But these changes were good for cleanliness and organization. I've learned that most kitchens don't meet the highest standards of tidiness. Some are scary places from a health point of view, especially when it comes to safe gluten free cooking. Whatever goes on in the kitchen isn't a secret, even if you keep the door shut, because if food makes people sick, they're going to figure out that something in the kitchen wasn't right.

When going to a restaurant or someone's home to eat, seeing the kitchen helps us know what to expect regarding potential glutening. Even so, culinary mysteries prevail. Being transparent is important in any business or relationship today, especially food.

Organizing Your Kitchen

In order to cook gluten free successfully you have to start in the kitchen. Whatever is made in the kitchen can be healthy and delicious, or make somebody sick as a dog (what *does* that mean exactly?). A reputable cook cannot afford to prepare foods in ways that make people ill. I had to perform a bit of restructuring to make sure our kitchen was GF safe, but the changes improved our cleanliness, organization, storage, and product purchasing. The biggest changes occurred in our head, not in the kitchen. Certain products I used to consider staples are no longer allowed in this room.

We've learned that kitchens can be dangerous places for people with gluten intolerance in several ways. Not having the appropriate ingredients to cook with is a huge factor. Another issue is having the right ingredients, but letting them become contaminated during the cooking process. The third problem arises when food is adequately prepared but improperly served.

You probably know by now that direct or cross-contamination may occur when items that contain gluten com into direct contact with gluten free foods. This happens in food service preparation areas through contaminated cooking areas or surfaces. It can also occur when food service providers are not strict about limiting gluten exposure. Wheat flour allegedly can float in the air for up to a week, so particles may cling to food preparation areas or utensils without anyone suspecting a problem. Gluten particles as small as 20 parts per million have been known to adversely affect a person with gluten intolerance. That's why some folks with celiac disease worry about going to a pizzeria that says it serves gluten free pizza. They may have a gluten free crust, but if wheat flour is hanging in the air, will it land on their pizza? If pizzas are all cooked together in an oven in the same time, is there possible contamination there? These issues aren't easily solved.

Pots and Pans. In most kitchens it doesn't matter what you cook in, so long as you clean well afterwards. However, when it comes to creating a safe kitchen for people who have gluten sensitivities, pristine pots and pans are a big deal. Some have surfaces that are "seasoned" by what was cooked in them previously. If that previous meal contained gluten and the pots weren't properly cleaned, the pan may contain a light surface of gluten that ends up contaminating someone. Other pans may have small cracks or indentations in them where food particles get lodged and are hard to see and remove. And sometimes we just don't get all the leftover food out when the pans are washed, especially if we're relying on the dishwasher.

I find it easiest to reserve special pots just for glutened foods (like wheat pasta) and others only for gluten free grains. When my mom died, I sentimentally kept a few of the pans she loved to cook in. These had so many gluten-based foods cooked in them that there's no way they could ever be clean enough for me to feel safe serving Chris food. So I keep them to cook pasta and remember childhood dinners of long ago. Today, my gourmet kitchen is much better for safe cooking. We have a separate griddle for making GF pancakes or grilled cheese sandwiches. Having separate equipment isn't a big deal once you organize a system. Problems occur if someone else comes to cook in your kitchen—that's when you must be a watchdog.

Restaurants ought to do this, because if you go into a restaurant and ask for a gluten free meal, how can you know they're protecting you by using pots and pans reserved only for gluten free foods.

Skillets are especially difficult to clean well, especially if food adheres to the bottom of the pan. They require hand scrubbing before going into the dishwasher. Cast-iron skillets are famous for picking up the oils and foods cooked in them; some cooks merely wipe them out and don't like to scrub them hard to preserve that quality in the pan—which could be a nightmare for people with celiac disease. Pans treated with surface coverings that make them easy to clean seem even more questionable than the old stainless steel pans, because those surfaces can chip or wear away, causing gluten particles to cling. Because it's hard to predict what's safe, I recommend reserving a couple of skillets for your gluten free cooking—and also pie tins, cookie sheets, and muffin pans.

Silverware and utensils are another issue. They can usually be successfully cleaned in an effectively run dishwasher. The scrubbing cycles tend to knock off any unrinsed food and the heat tends to kill germs. The biggest problem for utensils seems to be spoons and spatulas used during cooking. Wooden spoons may be beautiful, but they are difficult to properly clean. Spatulas or colanders that have tiny holes in them may be harder to clean than smooth surface types, since food trapped in the little crevices is hard to remove. They may look fine to the naked eye, but closer scrutiny will show hardened bits of food—especially the sticky glutened foods.

We recommend using separate cooking utensils for gluten free cooking. You can buy a special color for these things, mark them with a permanent marker, and store them in a separate place for gluten free utensils and cutlery.

Measuring cups are sneaky utensils GF people often forget about. Again, you can avoid contamination by keeping a special set of cups for gluten free measuring.

Toasters and equipment. Electric appliances can be costly, but you will need a separate set for gluten free cooking. Imagine using the same toaster for regular bread and then popping in a piece of gluten free bread. The contamination factor is huge. The same things holds true for waffle irons—getting rid of all wheat tidbits to make it totally gluten free is difficult. A deep fryer used to cook breaded foods won't be safe, especially if the same oil is used. Only by having separate equipment, one for regular food and one for gluten free food, can you be sure the food you prepare is safe and uncontaminated.

General items such as blenders and food processors are difficult to clean, because their little blades are sharp and close together. Colanders are breeding grounds for contamination, since it's virtually impossible to clean them sufficiently after draining wheat pasta in them. You need two colanders—one for wheat pasta and one for the gluten free foods. Never use the same cutting board, especially a wooden board. Ceramic cutting boards can be cleaned and sterilized, but not wooden boards. Once a cutting board is used, put it in the sink to designate it needs thorough washing. Having a designated gluten free cutting board ensures that someone won't cut a bagel on a surface and then another person innocently comes along and cuts food for a gluten free person. Even items like can openers can be a breeding ground for contamination if they're used to open cans containing glutened products .

Food Preparation Areas

The surfaces on which you cook should be absolutely clean. Unless you're on the Food Network, most cooks don't take off every item off their counter and scrub it down before settling in to cooking. Kitchens can be messy places where flour and crumbs scamper into tiny corners where they can be blown across the room to other areas. Ideally, a kitchen should have two separate areas, one for gluten free foods and one for glutened foods. Without this separation, every kitchen has a risk for cross contamination.

Ideally, you should have separate pieces of equipment; different utensils and cutting areas; separate refrigerators, stoves, ovens, and microwaves; separate storage pantries and dish washing areas, and even separate dishes.

My kitchen isn't right for two separate food preparation areas, so we practice strict cleanliness. I am forever washing my hands and washing down the stove, counters, equipment and food preparation areas. Using paper towels is recommended because after you wipe something down you just throw them away. Cloth towels just spread the gluten around, especially if used more than once before laundering. Sometimes when I'm cooking I wonder if the cutting board can be safely used again, and if I have to wonder, I've come to the conclusion that I just shouldn't do it. When in doubt, toss a cutting board, knife or other object into the sink and use one you're certain is clean. This is especially the case in homes like ours where some of us are gluten intolerant and some of us love wheat bread, cookies, crackers, and noodles. You should never take for granted that a cooking area, utensil, or equipment is safe if there's any chance someone else in the family was using them.

Grills

Aluminum foil is a wonderful thing for outside grills because it allows you to make sure food is cooked on a clean, safe surface. When cooking inside, some folks use an entirely separate grill for gluten free items to avoid contamination.

Restaurant grills can be hazardous for people with gluten intolerance. For instance, some breakfast diners cook up a mess of home fried potatoes to serve. These are fine when seasoned with salt and pepper, but if the cook adds seasoned salt that contains gluten, you're in trouble. If the potatoes contain breading to increase crispiness, then cooking eggs nearby leads to cross contamination. Similarly, steaks cooked on the grill can be fine—it it's plain steak. When meats are marinated, many of these products are not gluten free, so a marinade may contaminate the surface of the grill, even though nothing besides meat was cooked on it.

I find grill cooking is easy at home when you have a system. Going out to eat at a steak house is usually safe because meats are most often cooked on meat-only surfaces. But if people are using grills to cook pancakes or pannini's, that's a different story—a story that requires separate but equal cooking strategies.

Hands

Food preparation is a tricky thing, and even if safe ingredients are used and food is prepared on clean surfaces, contamination will occur if the hands of the person preparing food have been tainted through contact with gluten. I keep a large container of soap beside the sink that I can tap with my wrist to dispense soap, and while cooking I wash my hands many times during the process. For drying your hands, paper towels are better than cloth.

The easiest way to make sure hands are safe in restaurants is for cooks to wear gloves and change them between dishes. It's great when you can see the chef actually preparing your food. Consider these two examples:

I ordered a salad at a sub and salad chain, informing the server it was for someone with celiac disease and had to be made in a gluten free manner. The worker understood not to put croutons on the salad, yet she failed to put on clean gloves. It took me a moment to realize she was making my supposed-gluten free salad with the same gloves she wore while making a submarine sandwich a few minutes earlier. Even though the worker had gloves on, the bread particles were still present, and were passed on to the veggies she grabbed while making the salad. I told her I couldn't accept the salad she was making, and would she mind starting over with clean gloves? She was annoyed. She threw out the partially made salad in a huff, and aggressively tossed new greens and vegetables into a clean bowl.

Why couldn't she smile and say, "Oh, I'm sorry. I didn't realize what I was doing. Thanks for teaching me about that." Because of her huffy attitude, I never went back.

Now for comparison, consider a trip to 5 Guys for lunch. After placing my gluten free order, the staff shouted out to each other, "Gluten allergy!" and a preparer was assigned to just our order. He immediately put on fresh gloves. Their actions and attitude conveyed that they handled gluten free orders all the time, and they gave us pleasant conversation—not annoyance. They wrapped each of the food items separately to avoid contamination. This business has a policy that protects people with gluten sensitivities. We even watched the gloves get switched.

When a kitchen is behind closed doors, however, you can never be totally sure. The manager has to create a policy and monitor the workers to make sure glove procedures are followed.

The Oven and Cooking Surface

It's common to bake a pie or other food that spills onto the bottom of the oven. Every time the oven is used afterwards, the spilled food burns off, a little at a time. This means a glutened substance may lurk there long after the contaminating dish is removed and consumed. Ovens must be regularly cleaned, and ideally a separate oven is available for gluten free baking. Frankly, I don't clean my oven thoroughly as often as I should and we've never had a problem with cross contamination. But I think this is only because I don't cook a lot of wheat products that spill onto the floor of the oven. When they do spill, I immediately scrape it out.

Sometimes cooks will put glutened and gluten free foods into the same oven to bake at the same time—a formula for disaster. Because I only have one oven, in my early days of GF cooking I used to do this. I would have two pans of muffins (one glutened and one gluten free) and tuck them both in the oven at the same time to cook, so they would come out at the same time. Why did I think the gluten free muffins wouldn't be impacted? Now I cook the gluten free muffins first, then cook the foods with gluten. I check for spills afterward that I can quickly clean up.

When foods cook on top of the stove, it's normal to stir them and put the spoon nearby for later use. If the spoon is put down in the same spoon holder as one that has gluten on it, the GF spoon may become contaminated. It's also easy to forget what spoon was used in which dish and the wrong spoon gets plunked into a dish, so be careful! Sometimes lids that cover pots may be moved from one dish to another, which is a problem when a lid covering a glutened dish gets moved to a dish that needs to be gluten free. Particles may cling to the inside of the lid, and drip into the GF dish. When serving directly from the stove, make sure to have the gluten free foods placed on the back, not the front, so glutened foods or broths don't accidentally drop into a dish and contaminate it.

Dishwashing Recommendations

Before putting any dishes into the dishwasher, everything should be washed in soapy water to remove as many food particles as possible. Rinsing and scrubbing your dishes is essential, especially for items that have had bread, wheat pasta, or gluten in some form crusted on them. Imagine what happens to the entire load of dishes if a pan or plate smeared with glutened food is washed with plates people with gluten intolerance will eat from: Everything in the dishwasher could be contaminated. When taking clean dishes out of the washer, I often find a string of spaghetti lingering on a glass or bowl that never held the product. The excuse, "But I ran the dishwasher," just won't wash when it comes to cross contamination.

A good dishwasher is a vital piece of equipment in any kitchen. When washers run effectively with plenty of antibacterial soap, the powerful water jets wash away food remnants and the heat cycles kill any remaining germs. Some food preparers address the issue of cleanliness by never running pots and pans with plates, silverware, and glasses. This helps keep residue from cooking pots off the surface of plates, or lurking in the bottom of glasses. Make sure to clean the dishwasher bottom from time to time, just to make sure nothing weird has fallen underneath the rack that gets tossed up during a wash cycle.

Food Storage Areas

We have a cabinet dedicated to gluten free products, another cabinet just for wheat cereals, crackers, flowers, and pastas, and the largest cabinet for foods that are safe for everyone to eat. Keep gluten free products in separate cabinets, refrigerators, or storage areas. It's so much easier to store foods this way, because you know what to grab when you're in a hurry. Storing foods in designated places from the beginning and then returning them immediately after cooking makes preparing GF food much safer and more predictable. This simple organizational strategy is also helpful when people who aren't familiar with gluten free cooking come to help. They'll immediately know where to look for items and what they should avoid. Gluten free flour should never be kept alongside wheat flour; merely by sitting next each other, particles may "puff" when picked up or put down on the shelf. Particles of wheat flour may become airborne and land on gluten free products. Keeping the dry products, as well as the jarred and refrigerated types, in separate areas ensures all foods will remain safe until you use them.

Foods that come in jars, like peanut butter, jam, or mayonnaise, pose a special GF concern. It's easy when making a sandwich to put in a clean knife the first time and then decide you'd like a little bit more and put the knife back in for a dab, all without realizing the knife momentarily came into contact with bread. That's why we take a marker and write GF on the top of lids, so we know when it's safe to double-dip and when it isn't safe. This isn't a big deal once you get into the mindset of "look before you dip." The same is true of soft foods like butter and cream cheese that may be spread on breads. We keep the "gluten" cream cheese and butter in one area and store cream cheese and butter marked "gluten free" in another. Only one swipe of a contaminated knife can taint these foods.

Serving Food

Nothing is more frustrating than going out of your way to make a super gluten free dish, only to have someone contaminate the food before it reaches the table. Sometimes this happens by accident, like when RePublic waitress Holly plunked down wheat bread strips on a gluten free appetizer and dip. A sprinkle of croutons looks nice on a salad, but with a sweep of a hand a food that was safe suddenly isn't. You can't just pick the croutons off and assume the salad is okay. It won't be. Those little particles of bread got on the lettuce and fell into the bottom of the bowl, letting teeny gluten molecules that are invisible to the eye came into contact with parts of the salad. The five-second rule doesn't apply here—even if the croutons were only there for a few seconds, they could still someone sick. A brand new salad that has never been touched by the croutons must be made. If a wheat biscuit is placed on the plate of a gluten free entrée by mistake, it's too late. You can't pretend it didn't happen, or hope no one will find out. It must be thrown out or served to someone else who can eat gluten; and an entirely new entrée must be created. For people with minor gluten sensitivities, that little contact with gluten may not matter, but for others, it may matter a lot.

In another example we confront regularly, people will use a spoon in more than one dish to serve themselves. We're not trying to be anal, but we've learned to use the serving spoon that is in the dish and no other. If a serving spoon was used in the wheat based macaroni and cheese and then used to take a few peas out of another bowl, the peas suddenly become unsafe for anyone with gluten or lactose issues. Cafeterias, pot luck dinners, and buffets are hard to control. Likewise, at a frozen yogurt store the strawberries should be safe to put on top, but if people double dipped the spoon that also was in the cookie crumble topping, the strawberries are no longer safe and the innocent customer who comes in an hour later may never know.

Summary

When people go gluten free, usually kitchens are designed to have a small GF section, while the rest of the room is deemed unsafe. This means one part of the counter is GF safe, only a few pans or dishes are for-sure safe, and the person who is gluten sensitive is always under pressure to check that things are okay. What if you switched that model around? What if most of your kitchen was safe for everyone, with a small section just for gluten foods and gluten cooking? This is what we've done.

Our cabinets are all safe. Our dishes and pots and pans are generally safe for anyone who grabs a pan and starts cooking. I have a few pots and pans put aside to use for gluten cooking, but they are not in locations where people would normally grab them. For instance, I don't use the same pot to boil gluten pasta and gluten free pasta, even if I've washed it in between. Likewise, I use different muffin pans, even though I always use paper muffin cups in both. There is one colander for GF pasta and one for wheat pasta. I keep them in separate spots. Our counters are clean for cutting and regular use by everyone. I have one section of the counter I use when I'm making gluten things. I've located it in the most out-of-the-way spot to avoid the possibility of accidental cross-contamination.

The way we lay out our kitchens conveys who is important. Parsing out of tiny, out-of-the-way specific areas for gluten free cooking symbolically conveys the message, "You are different, you are weird, and you must be careful because you don't fit in with the rest of us." Frankly, it's discriminatory. If we value inclusion, then let's think about making kitchens safe for everyone. There are power differentials in the way we organize our kitchens. That's something important for you to think about.

Countless things in a kitchen can accidentally contaminate someone who needs a gluten free meal. All of them are preventable. Most of the steps to ensure safety are the same steps we should be using anyway. Cleanliness and protocols make food safer for everyone. And you know, once you organize your kitchen, gluten free cooking is easy—really, truly easy.

Chapter 4
Attitude Is Everything

HOW DO YOU FEEL about going gluten free? How about cooking for someone who's gluten free? Attitude is half the battle. In the pages that follow we'll talk about the attitudes of people who go GF, those who cook for them, and those who serve them.

When wheat-loving Chris first figured out he could never again eat Grandma's homemade bread, his favorite cherry criss-cross crust pie, or my from-scratch noodles, depression hit and he felt going gluten free was almost a fate worse than death. Like Chris, we all have a relationship with food that goes beyond what we like or dislike. Often, we're attached to the memories associated with eating certain foods, and these are hard to release.

Food is a big deal for most of us—having enough of it, and making it nutritious, attractive, and tasty. I felt like a culinary failure when I started trying to cook gluten free. My early attempts didn't taste good or look attractive; they were expensive to prepare, and we weren't sure about the nutrition. I relied on packaged foods none of us wanted to eat. At that point, cooking stopped being fun and eating became a dreaded chore. Menu construction was a struggle. Going out to eat was impossible. We were relegated to eating bad food at home and thinking we could never again go out to dinner and enjoy beautiful, delicious meals. We had a sense of lack about going gluten free. No wonder so many people think going gluten free is a genetic punishment.

To be honest, I'm not sure exactly what changed our attitude. Maybe it was access to new food products that came on the market; corn pasta certainly was a marked improvement over the slimy rice versions. Maybe it was getting better at cooking GF. Maybe it was because we saw the health benefits of limiting carbohydrates and gluten. But I think the biggest thing that changed us to liking GF was when we gave up on trying to substitute gluten and keep our old culinary lifestyle. We discovered it was entirely possible to eat well without any pasta or bread at all.

Cutting our addiction to bread type products meant we had to find different dishes to eat. And guess what? They were delicious and healthy for us. Meats, salads, and vegetables can be fixed in attractive and creative ways; rice is safe, and we use that as a staple when we want something for a base, as in Indian or Chinese food. Thin, clear rice noodles were amazing in our Pad Thai; corn tortilla shells made Mexican dishes more authentic and yummier than using wheat tortilla shells. My salads are scrumptious and it would be hard find a more delightful meal anywhere at any cost.

This evolution took time. At first we cooked gluten free just for Chris; he ate those products while the rest of us dined on regular pasta or bread on our sandwiches. This was for two reasons—the GF products cost more, and the food didn't taste good to his siblings, who turned up their noses at GF dishes in favor of "regular" ones. Chris felt like he was quarantined. We ate together, but we weren't eating the same things. Today, as a family we all eat a GF diet without blinking or complaining because there's nothing to complain about. The food is delicious. We extended our culinary repertoire as we learned what to buy, where to shop, and how to avoid cross contamination.

We also figured out that *what* we ate was less important than eating together. We eat food to live, not live to eat food. So if we have an enchilada made with corn instead of a flour shell, that's okay. It's better to eat together than have separate dishes that isolate the person eating gluten free. When we go out to eat now, we make sure there are safe foods for Chris to order, and we can all have whatever we each want at the same time. This may not seem like a big deal for most people, but when you've got dietary restrictions, it's a huge issue.

Think About What Happens When You Gluten People

As a general rule, we human beings are only concerned with things that directly affect us. When it comes to preparing food for people with gluten sensitivities, we wish other people realized that being glutened is a miserable experience for those who get sick. Seeing someone you love get sick because another person was careless is upsetting. Showing you care is important in any relationship.

Glutening people leads to hurt feelings. I remember accidentally glutening Chris because I wasn't being careful enough about reading the ingredients and how I prepared the food. Bottom line—my inattention to detail made someone I love terribly sick. That is forgivable, but it didn't need to happen. Even if glutening is an accident on the food preparer's part, it creates issues of trust and confidence for the person who got glutened.

One night a group of family and friends went out for a birthday celebration at The Melting Pot—a fondue restaurant whose manager assured us they could prepare gluten free broth, sauces, meats, and vegetables. We felt confident that a happy birthday dinner would result. Nope. Now, the restaurant did their share to make eating out a safe and pleasant experience. The pot of their classic bread-and-cheese fondue was placed at the far end of the table away from Chris to avoid a problem. Unfortunately, in the excitement of the evening and chatter around the table, someone innocently put a skewer with a bread hunk into the broth that was used for vegetables. That two-second slipup made the broth pot inedible for Chris. The person who made the slipup felt terrible, but what's done was done. She was embarrassed and accepted responsibility, but naturally felt a little defensive. While Chris understood it was an accident, it was frustrating because he now couldn't eat that dish. Ordering a replacement would take a while and felt like an inconvenience. The biggest issue was that Chris felt the slipup was a sign that the dipper didn't care enough to exert caution on his behalf. We have to remember innocent mistakes can produce an emotional response. Heads and hearts reside in different places; hearts are closer to the belly, which may account for why food has such an emotional component to it.

Being glutened is a miserable experience. The reaction can happen two ways. Sometimes people get sick immediately after ingesting gluten. Their stomachs become uncomfortable, sweats begin, and they head to the bathroom with cramps or diarrhea. I knew a woman who felt so bad she lay down on the dirty bathroom floor because she felt she couldn't stand up. When such a severe and fast reaction occurs, it's easy to tell what caused the problem. In other cases, people may not realize they've been glutened until the food passes through their intestines.

With a delayed reaction, it's harder to prove you've been glutened, especially to a defensive restaurant manager. In one case, Chris had a reaction from one of two restaurants. He didn't get wiped out like he does with eating glutened foods; the signs were more like what he gets from cross-contamination. We called the luncheon restaurant (where we had dropped a large amount of money for a fancy meal), and the manager assured me it couldn't possibly be their doing. The other restaurant said the same thing. But one of those places served food in a way that "got him." We didn't want to make a fuss, we just wanted them to know their kitchen procedures resulted in Chris getting sick and they needed to be more careful, especially if they ever wanted us to come back. Their responses were classic NIMBY (not in my back yard), a shirking "not me" reaction and a blaming attitude of, "you must have eaten something from somewhere else." Neither restaurant offered to make things right; no money back, no gift certificate so we could try them again, just the unleashing of the attack dogs. These places got our money that time but if they wanted us as return customers, they didn't do anything to ensure that.

For those of us who care, it's embarrassing and upsetting to cook something that makes someone else sick. However, most people aren't attentive to food allergies unless we have a wake-up call in our lives. I once took cream of pumpkin soup to a Thanksgiving dinner and someone asked me it the soup contained milk. My response was, "Just a little milk." Actually, I made the soup with a hefty amount of cream, plus butter. I didn't understand how "a little" of something could make another person sick, and I thought perhaps they wouldn't notice. I failed to understand what can happen when someone who is lactose intolerant eats lactose laced food. This wasn't lack of concern on my part—it was sheer ignorance.

For food service businesses, ignorance is not an acceptable excuse. Food establishments need to be aware of special diets and either accommodate them, or make it clear that certain diets can't be honored. This is basic customer service: Don't make your patrons sick.

Patrons today know their rights and they are not happy when slip ups occur. In our litigious society, getting sued is a real possibility. If someone tells you they're allergic to a food and you serve it to them anyway, they have a right to be annoyed. If you're a business and haven't been attentive to their needs, they may come after you for compensation. If you're going to serve gluten free foods, then do it right. If you are not, then put out a disclaimer that you don't, and you won't be held responsible. The biggest problems lie in the netherworld where you say you will, and then you don't.

If someone gets sick from eating in a restaurant, the manager needs to figure out what's going on. First, an internal investigation with an incident report will help the restaurant uncover possible contamination issues they were unaware of. Did a specific food trigger the problem, or did someone on the staff overlook gluten precautions? Did the event happen at a particular time, such as a busy Mother's Day when the kitchen staff was franticly turning out meals, or at particular hour of the day? By keeping reports, the manager can observe trends, such as a particular customer who complains regularly; a certain shift that has issues; or an employee who isn't following the guidelines.

When we take responsibility for feeding others, we also assume the responsibility for doing it safely. Choosing quality products is essential. Serving them well is important. And learning to proactively address gluten issues in the kitchen is vital. When dining problems occur—and they will sooner or later—the afflicted person wants is to know that people are sorry, they tried to make things right, and they will take measures so it won't happen again.

Changing the Attitude of Food Servers

Chris and I have met awesome food servers, hosts, and friends who bent over backwards to make sure he had a positive eating experience. For instance, his friend Jess searched gluten free recipes to find dishes that are delicious and pleasing to him. She spent hours decorating cookies, cakes, and creating dishes that were beautiful and amazing just because she's his friend. She even introduced us to gluten free products, such as the GF King Arthur's flour products. Her effort to meet his dietary needs endears her to us all the more.

At our favorite restaurants, members of the wait staff always remember Chris has special dietary needs. Instead of groaning, they seem excited to see us and happy to please us by ensuring his order is perfect. These people make us feel warm and happy inside.

For a restaurant, having a host and staff members who are responsive to food sensitivity issues will pay off in spades. People choose restaurants where their emotional needs, as well as hunger needs, are met. Studies show that customers purchase products they like from people they like rather than purchasing products they like from people they don't like (Mitchell 2011). Mitchell observed that front-line staff are often trained to be impersonal, efficient, rigid, and policy-oriented in the name of customer service, instead of being friendly and likeable. Dwivedi (2011) advises business people to be customer-centric, with individual needs at the heart of any decision. Good things start to happen when someone designs a business model around the customer.

We are advocating for a wholesale change in attitudes toward people with special dietary needs. We want hosts, whether at home or in restaurants, to treat people with food allergies thoughtfully, like normal human beings. Just because we need to avoid certain foods doesn't make us freaks. Don't snarl at us because we make your life inconvenient by asking for special food.

Consumer trends in the restaurant industry are evolving, and a smart restaurant will be aware of this, whether they like the trends or not. According to Gallup research of 25,000 consumers (O'Boyle 2011), about 46 percent of Americans spend less today than they did a year ago, and 35 percent of these people don't anticipate spending more in the future. The study found two important things – 1) spending is down significantly in both fast food and casual dining establishments, and 2) customer engagement, or the level of emotional attachments customers have with a restaurant and staff, is the highest predictor of where people go and how much they spend.

A Gallup study found that most consumers want more engagement from restaurant staff, even with fast food and casual dining. This is a heads-up to restaurant owners who should be more attentive to consumer needs. Exceptional customer service must address human interaction needs by helping customers feel genuinely cared about. Customers who feel welcome and appreciated are more likely to become loyal to the restaurant, visit more often, spend more, tip better, and become your ambassadors within the community (O'Boyle 2011).

Going out to eat is about more than food—it's about the experience. Restaurants that create positive dining experiences have been found to both engage customers and boost their wellbeing, both of which motivate customers to come again.

We found this was true when we visited Five Guys, the hamburger chain. The first time we stopped at one of their restaurants was an act of desperation after we'd been on the road for hours on a trip and were starving. Trying to find a gluten free restaurant at 9 p.m. was a challenge, and we had emotionally prepared ourselves to lower our standards. A Five Guys was right off the exit, so we decided to give it a try. To our amazement, the staff acted like our gluten free request wasn't a big deal, and they were delighted to fix our meals. The food was delicious and we were thrilled with the overall experience. So delighted, in fact, that when we got home we looked to see if any Five Guy restaurants were near us.

We found one close to home and went there in hopes of having another pleasant dining experience. We did! The second location offered the same high quality food, attentive staff, and enthusiasm. Now we know the people who work there and they always make us feel special. Their kitchen is organized so gluten free is no issue. Not only that, we can see everything that's done to the food. The meat has no fillers and is the only thing cooked on the grill. The buns are kept separate. The fryers only have fries in them, so no possibility of cross contamination with things like chicken fingers or onion rings, which they do not serve. Each burger dish is made on clean sheets of aluminum foil. The only thing a food preparer has to do differently for us is put on a clean pair of gloves and then make sure to have no contact with a bun. They wrap each item separately so we can put the burger together the way we want. They use gluten free brands of ketchup and mustard, so we have no problems with gluten even at the condiment level. We are regulars because we get treated well.

What to Look For

We're happy when we go to a restaurant and the staff makes eating gluten free a non-issue. We don't feel as though we're inconveniencing them, nor do they give us attitude. In short, they treat us like normal people making a reasonable request. On the other hand, it's a bad sign if the waiter gets a deer in the headlights look when we mention gluten, or acts annoyed when we ask questions about the food.

Over the years we've decided that management attitude is the biggest factor in how we're treated (Mindbiz.com 2011). If managers send out the attitude that gluten free options are important and can be easily implemented within the restaurant, successful GF policies and practices will naturally emerge. If an owner believes GF isn't important, the staff will follow his lead.

We love when restaurants put themselves in our shoes and convey the message that they are sensitive to gluten issues. How do they show it? Let's count the ways:

Check the menu. Are gluten free alternatives offered on the menu? Too often, salad is the only food item people with gluten sensitivities see on menus. Salads, as tasty as they can be, get boring. We want to see menu choices beyond the obvious.

Are gluten free items easy to identify? Are they listed on the menu so we can easily find them?

Are ingredients listed so we can see for ourselves what's being used? People with food allergies look for information to help them make safe selections. Even if the ingredients aren't on the menu, the wait staff should have access to the chef's recipe so we can find out what's in a dish when we ask. Chains like McDonalds provide this information on their websites and on a poster available for public review.

Do the menu dishes have **interesting names and enticing descriptions** that make us want to try them? If a menu lists only the names of food, it's hard to justify why a BLT in one restaurant costs so much more at one place than another. We like it when the picture of a scrumptious-looking BLT sandwich is located beside a description that reads something like this:

> Crispy slices of Vermont maple-cured bacon are nestled with locally grown luscious leaves of organic Romaine lettuce and sun-kissed, vine-ripened ruby-red Italian plum tomatoes. The delicious gluten free bread is freshly made by the Loaves of Plenty bakery here in our community, since we believe in supporting local establishments, and toasted to perfection. We make our own zippy mayonnaise to give you an extraordinary BLT experience. And of course, no gluten products or preservatives are ever used in our sandwich.

Ambience is always important. We may want to go to a coffee shop, an elegant restaurant, a fun pizzeria, a pub or sports-bar theme, or a hipster, trendy, happening place. While stereotypes indicate we can't trust sports bars as much as "green" establishments, Wild Wings wins hands down for their GF attentiveness.

Summary

The most important thing to remember as you leave this chapter is that if you're gluten free, it's a part of your life that has serious ramifications and you are responsible for figuring out how to make it work. That means you have to dig for information. You must be an advocate for yourself, because so many people don't understand the issues.

Even your friends and family members may think, erroneously, that if you're gluten free you're just catching the wave of a fad and a little gluten won't hurt you. A few folks think it's all in your head and they'll just slip contaminated food to you and you won't know. Our neighbor Laura has health issues she thinks will improve if she goes gluten free, but if she eats a little of it she won't get sick. For Chris, that isn't the case. Cooking in a pan that wasn't thoroughly cleaned from wheat pasta is just asking for trouble; picking off croutons before serving him a salad will make him sick because the crouton contaminated the lettuce. Almost always, Chris' body knows the truth.

Sometimes people aren't careful enough because don't understand gluten free issues, and sometimes they just don't care. But if they were one the unfortunate souls who get sick as a dog from gluten, I assure you—they'd learn to care.

If family or friends are not sensitive to your GH issues, the message is that they don't care. This is tough to accept. Even when people are caring in other ways, when they don't make the time and effort to make sure you have a pleasant dining experience, you won't like them as much. This is especially important in intimate interpersonal relationships.

Chapter 5
Dining Out

EATING OUT HAS BEEN our biggest challenge in going gluten free. We mastered the challenges of what to cook, how to cook, and where to shop. But going out to dinner? Not so easy. First we'll look at the issue surrounding dining out, then the types of eating establishments you routinely encounter and what you can expect from them. Finally, we'll explore other types of dining out, including catered events, camps, parties, school, and business meetings.

The Dilemmas of Dining Out Gluten Free

Dining out should be fun, but that isn't always the case for people who are going gluten free, especially at first. One time of being glutened by a restaurant is all it takes to make someone with celiac disease decide to stay home. When Chris gets sick, the effects can be immediate, awful, and lingering. Being seriously glutened makes him incapable of functioning for at least a day. He can't work, drive the car, or do normal chores. Imagine your head pounding, sweat pouring, and your guts on a roller coaster, flying from one extreme to another while you hold on for dear life, wondering how long the ride is going to last. Even in its milder forms, gluten intolerance feels like you're muddling through an amorphous fog, with no tangible symptoms you can put your finger on. Who on earth would want to go out to eat and risk this kind of result?

For a long time Chris shrugged with frustrated resignation and said it was easier to forgo the fun of going out to dinner to stay at home where he knew he could eat and be healthy. This was a wise choice, given the options we had available, but his decision impacted our entire family. The rest of us, who could eat gluten and didn't have to worry about getting sick, would either stay home and feel a bit sad because we couldn't go out to eat, OR we'd leave Chris at home alone while the rest of us when out for a fun dining experience. We would isolate him for food? Somehow that didn't seem fair. If he went to places where he didn't dare order anything, he had to sit there sipping a soda while everyone else enjoyed their meals.

By now, all of us have learned to scan menus, size up cleanliness, and assess the competence of waiters, cooks, and managers in order to decide whether a restaurant is safe. We're all excited when we find a place everyone can enjoy.

Going out with friends is hard when you're GF, because most people don't understand the gluten issue. Most young people like to eat at high-gluten places that serve pizza, burgers, fries, or beer. Chris can go, but he's pushed to the margin because he can't do what everyone else is doing. That is tough for a young person. Friends with young children realize they can't eat the cupcakes classmates bring to share for their birthdays; they can't run up to vendors at the amusement park and run off with a hotdog. When you can't eat what everyone else is having, you feel left out.

As one of the founders of Sociology of Food, I know that eating is an important factor in any human exchange. Food is social and symbolic as well as nutritious. We should be transparent in food preparation. The people who feed us should be friendly, efficient, thoughtful, and attentive to detail. Generosity of spirit is more important than generous portion size.

Why People Go Out To Eat

Celebrations

Social gatherings

No time to cook or prepare food

Nothing in the house to fix

Boredom/Entertainment

Wanting to be pampered

Hunger

Each of the reasons for going out is accompanied by anxiety for people who have food allergies. Friends and family members can help reduce our angst by helping ensure we won't get sick if we eat with them.

When people invite us to their homes for dinner, we appreciate having them ask if we have dietary needs or restrictions. That simple question opens a door to the conversation of what we can eat and what will make us sick. It sets the stage for a positive experience for everyone.

Restaurants are a prime concern for people who eat gluten free. A study by St. Sure (2011) identified that going out to eat evokes a variety of emotions for people who need carefully crafted meals in order to stay healthy. These include:

Anxiety over finding something they can safely eat.

Nervousness over whether they will be treated well and not get sick as a result of the meal.

Fear of being sick. Unless you've been sick from being glutened, you may not appreciate how intense this fear and concern may be.

Awkwardness whether they can dine out with others and not be perceived as annoying.

Embarrassment. Getting sick may force someone to leave the table for an extended time and hover in the bathroom over the porcelain throne. Some restaurant bathrooms leave much to be desired.

Regret and sadness. Having to watch every single morsel that passes your lips is annoying and can make a person sad. Everyone else seems to be able to eat whatever they want. Sometimes the "Why me?" moment occurs unexpectedly.

Anger or resentment. While some people experience just regret or sadness over having to eat a restricted diet, others grow angry and resentful. These negative emotions can lead to volatile situations with others. If someone gets glutened from eating with you, there's a chance their anger will be directed at you.

Hunger if someone is famished and can't find anything to eat (except perhaps a boring salad). We've often left the table still feeling hungry.

Dining in Restaurants

How do we find gluten free menus when we go out to eat? We usually depend on word of mouth, the internet, and social media. More and more restaurants are advertising gluten free menus, mostly because they want to be on board to meet consumer demands. All restaurants are not equal. Some of these places do gluten free well, while others are questionable and offer only one or two safe items.

Google began tracking gluten free restaurants over the past few years when their search engine showed massive growth in searches for gluten free dining (Glutenfree.com – March 2010). The demand for this kind of information has at least doubled in the last two years, which goes to show the tide is turning as gluten free eating edges into the mainstream.

We live in a town with fewer than 4000 people and two dining establishments—one that offers breakfast and lunch and one offering lunch and dinner. I can list virtually every item on their menus from memory, and I know there's only one for-sure gluten free item—a GF pizza the dinner place recently began offering. Everything else in both places is a risky. The town north of us has three restaurants: a fish-n-chips place we suspect isn't safe, a Mexican place that could have been

GF but wasn't and made him sick, and a steak pub that is safe only if Chris orders a plain steak and baked potato. The dearth of options forces us to go farther afield when we want to have a nice dinner out.

We know it's a challenge to be familiar with all eating establishments, especially if you don't live near them. And new menu items appear all the time, even with fast food restaurants.

That's why we rely on social networking, where people with gluten issues share a bond and help one another.

People who need to eat gluten free are always on the look-out for information about where to go and where to avoid. Some of the most commonly used restaurant review sites include Yelp, Zagat, Urban Spoon, Gayot, Top Table, Restaurantica, Fodors, Dine.com, Open Table, Trip Advisor, Restaurant Row, or Menu Pages. Social media is a lifeline for gluten free diners, because happy customers are glad to tell others about their wonderful dining experience—and unhappy customers want to protect other diners.

You'll find thousands of guides for gluten free restaurants on the internet. Here are the most popular:

- *Find Me Gluten Free:* http://www.findmeglutenfree.com/ At this user-friendly site you can put in your zip code or name of town and find nearby restaurants that proclaim to have GF foods.

- *The Gluten free Registry*: http://glutenfreeregistry.com/ - A searchable, online database of over 16,400 restaurants, bakeries, caterers, groceries, and other "gluten free friendly businesses" throughout the United States.

- *A Gluten free Guide to Restaurants*: http://aglutenfreeguide. com/restaurants - This site provides extensive lists of national restaurants chains that claim safe, gluten free menus. They also have a list of establishment in New York, the United States, and a variety of international locations.

- *The Gluten free Restaurant Awareness Program* (http://www.glutenfreerestaurants.org/) provides an online searchable database of restaurants that participate in the restaurant-education program operated by the Gluten Intolerance Group.
- Celiac.com http://www.celiac.com/ can help you identify restaurants and provides education about a variety of gluten issues.
- The 75 *Essential Gluten Free Restaurant Menus You Need to Know* guide categorizes restaurants by the cuisine they serve, so if you've got a hankering for Southwest fajitas, pub food, or almost any ethnic type, you'll know where to find gluten free dining. (Shortened link: http://dld.bz/d2tQK).
- Triumph Dining (http://www.triumphding.com) sells a series of books such as *The Essential Gluten free Restaurant Guide* that list gluten free restaurants. The books are frequently updated and are useful for finding the locations of gluten free restaurants and their offerings.
- Gluten free Living: The Reality of Navigating the Restaurant World. Posted by Gabby's Gluten Free - http://dld.bz/d2tQN (shortened link).

If people with gluten intolerance are traveling in countries where different languages may be dominant, it is important to carry a translation card that states you have a gluten allergy and need to have special procedures followed in preparing your food. Cards diners can provide to wait staff to explain their need for gluten free food can also be purchased at the website www.Celiebo.com. These cards come in English, Spanish, Hindi, Italian, Thai, Vietnamese, Arabic, Chinese, French, German, Japanese, and Greek. This requires planning ahead, but if you know you're traveling to an area where there is a concern about whether restaurants will prepare safe food for you, this is an option (Keller 2011).

If traveling, you may want to carry a doctor's note on you that states you have celiac disease or a disorder that requires a special gluten free diet. This may help offset problems for the traveler when requesting special attention to meal preparation. The Gluten free Travel Site. com at http://glutenfreetravelsite.com/ provides information to help consumers find restaurants, groceries, hotels, resorts, and cruise ships that accommodate gluten free diets. Their information is searchable by city or zip code and they have international as well as domestic sites. They also offer reviews from customers about their dining experiences. You'll also find hotel, resort, and restaurant reviews from people in the gluten free community.

Gluten Free Restaurant List

Many chain restaurants have identified being gluten free is the way to go. Upscale restaurants with chefs are often willing to create great gluten free dishes, even if none are listed on the menu. Some smaller independent, mom-and-pop type restaurants are safe, while others are not.

Certain gluten free products may cost a little more, and the cook and servers must exercise greater care in serving gluten free foods, so it makes sense that restaurants may charge more for gluten free foods. Most people who have to go gluten free are willing to pay the extra amount in order to be safe.

Even though the number of gluten free restaurants has increased, we frankly don't understand why so many other establishments fail to provide gluten free foods on their menus. If restaurants can't appreciate the moral and health imperatives of gluten freedom, then the sheer financial incentive should persuade them to go gluten free. Paul Antico, founder of AllergyEats, encourages restaurants to better accommodate diners with allergies, not only because it is the right thing to do, but it will also help them to make money: "Savvy restaurateurs understand the financial benefits of providing allergy-friendly environment... Many restaurant owners are wisely taking extra precautions to accommodate food allergic and intolerant guests, having their employees trained in allergy safety, creating gluten free menu options, providing ingredient lists, and seeking industry certifications" (http://bit.ly/1EzSgeG).

Restaurant chains that made the leap to serving gluten free fare include:

Applebees	Austin Grill
Biaggis	BJ's Restaurant and Brewhouse
Bonefish	Boston Market
Carrabbas	Cheeseburger in Paradise
Chili's	Five Guys
Fresh to Order	Garlic Jim's
Glory Days	Legal Seafood
Margarieta's Mexican Restaurant	Not Your Average Joe's
Old Spaghetti Factory	Olive Garden
Outback Steak House	On The Border
Paneras	P F Changs
Picazzos	Pizza Fusion
Rockfish Seafood Grille	Ruby Tuesday
Sam and Louie's	Subway
Ted's Montana Grill	Unos
Village Tavern	Wendy's
Wildfire	Z'Tejas Southwest Grill

These are just the tip of the iceberg. These restaurants have caught on to the fact that they need to diversify their menus because the customer base is diversifying. However, you need to be aware that each dining establishment varies in how they view gluten free. Some make it no big deal, while others seem clueless. Some restaurant staffers are thoughtful and helpful, while others are oblivious or rude. In the next section we've categorized the different styles of dealing with gluten issues.

Restaurant GF Styles

As gluten free consumers, we've encountered a full range of gluten free dining experiences, from wonderful to horrible. After years of dining out, we developed a quick-and-easy way to size up a restaurant so we know what to expect—and whether to stay or go.

Type 1: "It's Your Problem."

This type of establishment doesn't pretend to be gluten free. Staff members are relatively clueless, and the general rule is, "dine at your own risk." A perfect example is a popular local tavern in our community. They have a great bar with a wide range of alcohol offerings, including the best selection of beers in the state. With an ambiance reminiscent of a European pub, the tavern is tasteful, comfortable, and fun. They offer live music every evening and a variety of special events. This place is our Cheers. But as a family, we can never go there together unless gluten free family members will be satisfied drinking a ginger ale or club soda with lime. We've asked the manager several times if the restaurant has anything on the menu that is "safe," but they can't come up with a single acceptable food item. The closest thing would be a salad, but the kitchen is always so busy that cross-contamination is likely. They have no idea whether or not the dressings are gluten free.

While the manager and wait staff are nice, they clearly are NOT a gluten free establishment. This is something we figured out over time by communicating with the management.

The pros of this approach are straightforward. Be honest with customers up front, and if they decid to take a chance, the restaurant feels they're off the hook because they never promised anything. Unfortunately, this approach makes dining out difficult for people who need to go gluten free. These restaurants usually lose the entire population of gluten free consumers.

Type 2: GF R Us.

Unlike the pub described above, a few restaurants have chosen to be exclusively gluten free. They serve no gluten products, so zero chance of contamination. They have a limited number of dishes, but the menus tend to be healthy and delicious. Many gluten free restaurants are also sensitive to vegetarian, vegan, and lactose issues, plus other dietary concerns. Usually perceived as alternative establishments, they tend to be small and often have a funky ambiance. Everyone knows each other and the places are magnets for people with gluten issues. Some sell gluten free cooking products or take-home foods to supplement their restaurant food sales. These specialty restaurants are uncommon and often barely survive, because most people don't understand how delicious gluten free can be.

On the plus side, these restaurants are 100 percent safe from cross contamination and the food is healthy. Staff members are knowledgeable about gluten and other food issues, so the comfort level for consumers is high. The biggest problems for totally gluten free establishments is finding enough clients to pay the bills. Their smaller menus may be a turn-off for people with narrow perspectives of cuisine. Advertising can help, because the best way for them to survive is by getting the general public to come in and try their food.

One of our favorite gluten free only establishments recently closed; they couldn't make it financially when their rent went up. Having a larger, more regular customer base might have saved them. Their food wasn't overly expensive, seating was limited, and the atmosphere was rather Spartan in order to keep their costs down. Perhaps having a larger, nicer restaurant with more social things to offer would have helped them survive.

Type 3: All Talk and No Action.

This strategy is used by restaurants who want to seem as though they're sensitive to the needs of the gluten free diner, but aren't.

If a restaurant says they are not confident of serving gluten free food safely, we appreciate their honesty. The problem arises when they say they will—and then don't. We've had several dining encounters with restaurants who promote themselves as gluten free establishments, but aren't safe for people with celiac disease. Chris's body always knows—and so will yours.

One year on December 23, our clan gathered to celebrate by going out to dinner and then to the Palace Theatre. I stopped by the RePublic restaurant in advance to check it out, talk with the staff, and make sure they understood the importance of safe dining. They gave me a copy of their gluten free menu and assured me they were well equipped to deal with gluten free needs. Going there for our special holiday dinner seemed a safe bet.

When we arrived, Chris informed our server named Holly that he had celiac disease. She assured him everything would be fine. We ordered three appetizers from their gluten free menu. To our surprise, two of the dishes arrived on a plate surrounded by bread strips—not gluten free bread strips, but wheat. It seemed like a no-brainer to us that putting gluten products on top of gluten free food will cross-contaminate. Evidently the chef had prepared this dish properly, but Holly added the bread on top. Chris could only eat one of the appetizers.

Chris ordered his entrée from the gluten free section of the menu and selected the designated house favorite, steak and frites. The food was beautifully prepared and tasted great. But by the time we reached the theatre two-blocks away, he was already feeling the tell-tale signs of being glutened. He was sweating, his stomach and gut were rocky, and his head felt foggy. We settled into our front row, center balcony seats to watch the delightful performance, only to see Chris white as a ghost, clenching his hands together, trying to make it through the first act. While he did the stiff-upper-lip thing, trying not to spoil anyone else's evening, he couldn't enjoy the play. We didn't either because we were all worried about him. We left the play early to get Chris home where he spent the rest of the holiday between the bathroom and his bed, dealing with the physical distress of being glutened.

I phoned the restaurant and talked with the manager about the situation. Holly, he informed me, should have reported Chris' gluten needs to the staff when we first arrived. When she plated the food in such a way as to contaminate it, she should have immediately talked with the manager, brought a new safe dish, and deducted the contaminated food from our bill. He then admitted the fries listed on the gluten free menu were actually cooked in the same fryer as breaded items.

If an establishment promotes itself as gluten free, customers logically assume they know how to do it safely. Training matters. When customers get glutened, it's appropriate to apologize, give their money back, and otherwise make amends. When this didn't happen, we "helped" them learn how to serve GF safely by having the public health department pay them a visit.

All this misery was 100 percent preventable. It's one thing if a restaurant never promises to serve gluten free; it is quite another to say they do and then don't.

Type 4: "Read the Menu."

Type 1 restaurants don't pretend to be gluten free; Type 2 are only gluten free; Type 3 say they have gluten free items and assure you certain foods will be safe, but they are not. Type 4 restaurants make it clear they don't know whether they are gluten free or not. We've learned that many restaurants and waiters are clueless about what they serve from a gluten free point of view. When we state that someone in our party is gluten free, a glazed look passes over the faces of those who don't know, and they usually take one of two responses. One, the waiter admits he doesn't know and suggests we read the menu. However, few menus contain a detailed list of ingredients. Two, the waiter calls the manager or chef to have them explain what is, or is not, in the food.

This is actually a reasonable strategy, because if the manager marches into the kitchen to announce, "Table 17 has a gluten allergy," chances are the staff will pay attention, if for no other reason than fear of getting in trouble.

As a result, we've developed a refined ability to read a menu and ask key questions. Smart restaurants have notations on the menu that indicate which items are gluten free, vegan, etc. Most don't. So we look for items that should be safe, but may not be. We ask questions: "Are your mashed potatoes made from scratch or are they instant?" "Do you use your fryer for both breaded and unbreaded foods?" Knowing how to read a menu leads to intelligent conversations while ordering. If a waiter is perplexed by requests for more information about ingredients or cooking style, ask for the manager. If the manager looks confused, arrogant, or avoidant, just pack up and leave—the chances of being glutened are simply too great to risk.

We appreciate restaurants that proactively identify which foods are gluten free, vegan, or meet other specialized dietary needs. We look for the certified safe symbol or code. If the menu lists specific items that are gluten free, then everyone—customer, waiter, and chef—knows what to expect. This makes for clear communication. Listing the ingredients is also a good strategy. Asking questions of the staff provides them with a learning opportunity to assess how comprehensive their gluten free options really are.

Type 5: "We Serve Everything."

Some restaurants attempt to be all things to all people. This is understandable, given a tough economy where restaurants want to serve foods that appeal to everyone. For instance, a restaurant may offer steak, chicken, fish, and vegetarian dishes; Italian, Thai, Middle-Eastern, and Mexican dishes. They may list menu items that appeal to an expensive dining experience, alongside cheap finger foods that are quick to prepare and serve. We've learned that a complicated menu leads to a greater risk for gluten contamination. Food preparation surfaces may not be totally cleaned between food items, and a little smidge is all it takes to make someone quite sick indeed.

We know it absolutely IS possible to serve everyone. Countless restaurants prove this by proactively developing gluten free items on their menu. For example, the national chain Boston Market has a diverse menu that clearly notes food allergens of all types. Their menu and list are posted online and in their restaurants

Outback Steakhouse provides a gluten free menu with many options, so GF diners can share the same basic dining experience as their friends without issue. For fast-food, diners can eat safely at Wendy's, which offers salad, potatoes, chili, and dessert options for gluten free diners.

Smaller restaurants pose the biggest problem for eating gluten free in a "we serve everything" environment. This is especially true for kitchens with limited space in which to prepare and cook foods, but it can also be problematic for large chain restaurants. For instance, many pizza chains have introduced a gluten free pizza. But gluten free websites are quick to warn potential customers that wheat flour possibly floating in the air and contaminating the preparation surfaces and ovens can lead to cross-contamination. We're thrilled that restaurants are introducing gluten free products, but unless they properly prepare, cook, and serve the food, then customers should be wary.

Another possible problem is the food quality. Serving frozen items that are microwaved can allow a restaurant to offer many dishes, but most of these frozen, processed foods aren't as good as fresh, homemade dishes.

Non-restaurant Dining

If you're like most people, you dine in diverse places, including catered events, school, pot luck dinners, parties, and meetings. This can be extra challenging for people with gluten issues. We don't want to call attention to ourselves in a group setting, but we also don't want to end up sick.

As I've noted before, most people aren't trying to poison us—they just don't know any better. That's why it's important to educate the people you care about and the places you go. These suggestions are written for you—the gluten sensitive person—and for the servers, camp directors, cooks, and hostesses who will be feeding you.

Schools and child care facilities

Children with gluten intolerance are a concern for well-meaning teachers and school officials. Most school districts have multiple schools and use a single buyer and food preparation system—the days of the school lunch lady who actually cooked in the kitchen while the kids were in class are gone. This means gluten free diets need to be front and center throughout each school district, at all levels.

Many children have inherited gluten sensitivity that has not yet emerged into full-blown celiac disease. They may experience some of the symptoms, but not all. Doctors aren't quick to diagnose gluten sensitivities, and given the variety of symptoms associated with the disorder, it often takes a while for them to put everything together. Teachers and school nurses are in a unique position to see children who complain often of stomach pain or gastro-intestinal upsets. Hopefully, they will notify the parents when this becomes a regular occurrence and suggest a medical work-up. There isn't much a school or day care can do if a child has not been identified as having problems with gluten.

What schools *can* do is send out a nutrition survey at the beginning of the school year asking parents to identify whether their children have allergies or special dietary needs. Students with allergies of any sort can be culled from the list and put into a special consideration category for school nutritionists, food service workers, and teachers. Whether gluten or peanut, school personnel who act in loco parentis must know about each child's special needs.

Schools are faced with four major forms of food distribution issues: lunch, snacks, special events, and field trips. Each of these needs special consideration and collaboration with the parents.

Some schools and child care centers require students to bring their lunch and snacks. This gets the school off the hook for serving foods that aren't safe for the child, as well as increasing the chances that children will like, and therefore eat, their food. It also gives parents control over what their child will eat, and how much.

Many schools provide children with an option of buying school lunches. Usually, the menus are set weeks in advance by a school or district level nutritionist and posted somewhere for the children and parents to review them. But these menus don't include the ingredients, so parents and children have no idea what's actually in the foods. Proactive schools should post not only "what's for lunch," but also what's IN the lunch. A webpage with nutritional information is easy to create, and if all the students in a district are eating the same food, this would be a service to everyone.

It is possible to create allergy-free menus for students who need special consideration. The problem is, bread and pasta foods are inexpensive, fill up hungry kids, and children tend to like those foods. Schools don't like to cut these gluten foods from their menus. However, if the school knows about the allergy, they might keep gluten free substitutions available in the freezer and cook them shortly before the student's lunch period begins. In this way, a student with gluten allergy can still eat the same foods at lunchtime with his classmates, such as mac and cheese, pizza, or chicken fingers. There would be a cost differential, as gluten free foods tend to cost more. This cost may be willingly paid for by the parents, or perhaps by the district. The point is, school lunches can (and should be) created so that every child can safely eat them without feeling different.

Field trips often require students to eat away from school—and that's part of the fun. Dietary issues are easy to solve by asking each student to bring a bag lunch. This puts total responsibility on the student and parents. If students will be dining out while on a field trip, it's important to find the name and contact information of the eating establishment and provide that information to parents, along with probable costs. The parents can then contact the restaurant and find out if gluten free options are available. This strategy takes the pressure off school and puts the responsibility in the hands of the family.

Special events are challenging for a school, because students often bring treats such as cupcakes or cookies. At the beginning of the school year, a letter could go home from the teacher to all the parents indicating if any students have allergies that they should consider if they bring treats. Of course, it would not be appropriate for the teacher to identify information about which children have the allergies, although children tend to already know that. Hopefully, parents will be careful about sending foods all the children can eat, or providing alternatives for those with allergies. Plain popcorn, fruit, or veggie sticks are great options that are healthy for everyone.

But people love celebrations and sweets. Children hate being left out, and sometimes kids with gluten issues will eat foods that aren't safe for them so they won't feel left out. On the days when children bring in frosted cupcakes or chocolate chip cookies, it would be easy for a teacher to send an aide into the school kitchen's freezer and get a gluten free cupcake or cookie for the gluten sensitive child. The child wouldn't feel left out, the forgetful parent wouldn't be embarrassed, and life could move forward in a happy and harmonious way.

For this and other occasions, the school freezer could be stocked with a selection of cupcakes, muffins, cookies, pizza, or other food items that may be commonly shared at birthday parties or classroom celebrations. Having boxes of gluten free cookies or crackers in the cupboard wouldn't be expensive or inconvenient for the school. If your school system can't seem to manage this, perhaps they'll allow you, the parent, to place alternative frozen treats in the freezer, labeled with your child's name.

Sometimes children may not know if gluten is in a particular food item. Younger children may not have that information. Even if they ask, "is this food safe for me to eat?" others may not know, or infer a different meaning to the question and assure the child the foods are safe when they're not. Most of the time, the incorrect assurance is given out of ignorance.

Helping children learn to be sensitive about other people's health conditions can be an important way to teach tolerance and inclusion in the classroom. Providing tasty alternative foods for gluten free children will help others learn that different may not be bad or a big deal.

Refusing or neglecting to address the needs of a child with food sensitivities is a form of discrimination. At the very least, the child may feel left out. It can also become a source of teasing and aggression from other children. At worst, not meeting their needs can bring lawsuits.

The military

Any group that serves food to large numbers of people knows they're going to encounter food allergies. Organizations like the military serve thousands of people and are responsible for their health and well-being, both on the field and off. This includes making sure they have enough of the right foods that won't make them sick. Soldiers in the Army, Navy, Air Force, Marines, or other units who are contaminated with gluten are unable to perform their duties for a day or two. In fact, they pose a danger to their units and to themselves. It must be remembered that people who experience gluten intolerance may suffer from both physical and emotional problems that incapacitate them.

The Gluten Free Standards Association questions whether military administrators realize the impact gluten intolerance can have on soldier performance. It seems the new rise in gluten intolerance and the link to abdominal discomfort could change the Department of Defense's operating procedures on nutrition for our country's protectors. Celiac disease may disqualify someone who wants to serve and result in enlisted men and women being automatically discharged when diagnosed during their contract. The Department of Defense has not made a specific policy regarding gluten intolerance, but some members within the military are proactively addressing the issue of gluten problems. Allergens can be as deadly as friendly fire for people whose systems can't handle them.

Catered events

Weddings, birthday parties, anniversaries, retirement parties, conferences, rites of passage parties, showers or other celebratory events may be catered affairs. Caterers serve a special role because they serve a limited menu to a large number of people in a quick and efficient manner. These events pose special concerns for gluten free diners. We've learned to eat ahead of time when going to events where food is served, because we can't be sure that a) they will serve something we can eat and b) that even "safe" food won't get contaminated before we have it.

Catered events often sensitively provide gluten free foods, such as cheese, fruit plates, and veggie platters. If we're first in line to get these safe foods before too many other people take their share, we may be in luck. From a social point of view, rushing to the front of the line makes us look greedy. But the further we are back in the line, the greater the risk. People are well-meaning, but if a cheese platter is next to a cracker plate, you can be pretty sure someone will grab some crackers and pick up cheese with them, thereby contaminating all the other cheese pieces with gluten. Folks without gluten sensitivity simply have no idea how simple, mindless acts can influence others. The innocent guest who picked up glutened food with one fork may use that same fork to take food off a gluten free dish. People will use the same tongs to take a piece of bread and then a celery stick. People use crackers to swoop up a dab of hummus from the collective bowl, thereby rendering it unsafe for everyone. They may take a spoon designated for one food item and use it to serve another. Or they may do something as simple as scoop GF foods onto their plate, but the serving spoon touches bread or foods that contain gluten. Once this happens, even foods that should be safe suddenly aren't. This is like gambling—you never know what will happen, so the safest thing is to avoid eating. **Cross-contamination is a nightmare for gluten insensitive people when dining at cafeterias, salad bars, or congregant food-sharing events.**

We've learned to call ahead when attending a conference or wedding where dinner will be served to let the caterer know we need to have food especially prepared. The problem is, we can communicate with the caterer and feel comfortable our needs will be met, but when waiters come out with trays where over a hundred meals have been set up at once, we can't be sure of getting a totally safe plate. Contamination increases exponentially with the number of hands working with the food. Servers usually have no understanding of ingredients in the food they serve. These folks don't get much training, because the team of workers is different for every event.

Unless they contracted to provide gluten free foods, the caterer is under no obligation to do so. If a customer calls ahead of time to alert them to a dietary need, this is helpful because it gives the caterer a little time to come up with an alternative. If frozen gluten free foods are available, then they can be easily heated and served without a high chance of contamination, even when the wait staff is busy and not well-trained in the art of gluten free dining.

Having a person sit out the meal without eating doesn't look good for the hostess or the caterer. There are ways caterers can increase the chances that people with gluten allergies can eat safely, and it won't be too much extra work for them.

Menu Selection. Often caterers are confronted with patrons who want to put on an abundant spread without paying much. This is understandable, especially on constrained budgets. A wise caterer will educate their customers about the increasing number of people with food allergies, and the need to provide food everyone can eat. Caterers should offer menus that include meats, fish, vegetarian dishes, lactose free items, and gluten free options.

Guest pre-event food selection. Once a menu is set, the host may be able to send out electronic invitations where people can respond if they are coming, list their food choices, and speak up about special dietary needs. This lets the caterer know exactly how many people need special diets and who those people are. Sometimes the host can pre-seat guests so the servers know everyone at tables 7 and 11 have special diets. All too often, the host has no idea about the dietary needs of particular guests, so asking is an act of thoughtfulness.

Buffet Table Organization. Caterers often rely of buffets that allow people to serve themselves and select portion sizes. This is a problem for folks with gluten intolerance because no ingredients are listed and we can't always tell for sure what's safe. Posting a list of ingredients would be of significant help to all guests.

I do NOT recommend placing foods willy-nilly for ascetics or staff convenience. While it's common to organize salads in one area, entrees in another, and desserts in another, this old-school model doesn't address contemporary needs for dietary information. The easiest thing for a caterer to do is to have NO glutened foods on a special table, marked by sign that reads, Gluten Free. This simple method prevents cheese, fruit, cracker, dips, and other specially prepared gluten free foods from being contaminated by breads, crackers, or utensils that have touched glutened foods. Items like sautéd vegetables and roasted chicken breasts may be served in a separate area, apart from bread, pasta dishes, and other gluten foods.

Plated Catering. Some catered events call for a sit-down dinner. If this is the design, then the caterer needs to know who signed up ahead of time for gluten free meals. A thoughtful hostess will place a card on each table that announces, "Please notify your server of any allergies or dietary needs" to open the conversation between guest and server. A savvy caterer will keep extra gluten free and allergen-free food in a freezer. This shows great sensitivity on the part of the caterer and reflects well on the host.

We recommend that caterers use "safe" food items whenever possible, such as gluten free salad dressing everyone can enjoy. Salads can be gluten free merely by not adding croutons. Entrees are a matter of discussion, but it isn't hard to simply bake a chicken breast with butter, salt and pepper, have steamed vegetables, and a rice that doesn't use glutened seasonings (check to make sure, as gluten seasoning can sneak into rice products). Use butter in little packets or serve people individual containers of their own butter instead of having a shared butter stick or bowl everyone is putting their knives into. Put a basket of dinner rolls on the table, not on individual plates. Choose a "safe" dessert everyone can eat, such as ice cream that contains no cookie or gluten products, or fresh fruit with mint leaves. If cookies or cakes are served, then gluten free alternatives should be available. Whipped cream in a can will transform any dessert from mediocre to magnificent, especially when a gluten free garnish is used. It's easy to create an entire catered event with healthy, gluten free foods without anyone noticing the difference.

Wedding cakes and other special foods. Caterers know we enjoy certain foods as a form of social bonding. People who attend a wedding look forward to the cutting of the cake and eating a piece for good luck. Usually, wedding cakes are highly selected items and being gluten free is not one of the considerations. No problem. A smart caterer will have slices of lovely gluten free cake available at a separate, and identified, table so people who need gluten free food can also celebrate.

Transparency is key. If foods are presented in a safe manner with the ingredients posted, guests know the hostess cares about them. People with allergies who find nothing safe to eat will feel their needs don't matter, and that is a dangerous message for any hostess to send.

Summer camp

Going to summer camp is one of the joys of childhood—and so is eating. That's why being left out of camp cuisine is a huge disappointment. Every kid loves to make s'mores, but if you're a gluten free kid, you can't eat regular graham crackers, so all you can do is toast a marshmallow and bury it between squares of chocolate before everything melts.

As a parent, your job is to make sure the camp understands your child's needs and can meet those needs. Take care of this well in advance of opening day by using the intake forms and following up. Savvy camp directors know how to substitute appropriate foods, such as cookies and crackers, peanut butter and jelly sandwiches with gluten free ingredients, and gluten free spaghetti. Your child can make hot fudge sundaes, enjoy catching popcorn pieces in midair, and raid the kitchen at midnight for a snack without getting sick.

From the camp's point of view, this requires a) asking the right dietary questions of parents, b) working with the cook to create menus that work for everyone, c) purchasing special foods to keep on hand as needed, and d) making sure each camper feels normal, respected, and valued—just like the other kids. Food is symbolically important, and camp food can teach kids great lessons of inclusion.

A thoughtful dietician can construct allergy-free meals that are healthy, tasty, and full of the traditional camp experience. All it takes is a little planning.

Family, friends, and house parties

Basically, the guidelines for house parties are similar to catered events. A good host or hostess finds out about her guests' dietary needs and preferences, creates a menu to accommodate them, purchases the right foods, and prepares them in a safe way. The hostess should also serve food in a manner that limits contamination possibilities and double check with guests to make sure their needs are being addressed.

It is thoughtful to tailor the foods around the needs of those you've invited to be your guests. Gluten free folks aren't the only ones who have to watch what they consume. Some people are lactose intolerant, so creamy cheese and broccoli soup would be impossible for them to eat; a diabetic may have difficulties with the sugar-infused dessert; the guest who fights congestive heart failure may find the sodium-rich entree can create major problems later. Let's not overlook the Jewish guest who eats only a Kosher diet, the Muslim who eats a Halal diet, or the vegan who doesn't eat eggs, milk, or anything cooked with chicken broth.

In an example of tailoring a meal for gluten free guests, Maria was aware of the gluten issue and tried to fix a meal that would accommodate everyone. The problem was, she used the same pots and pans to cook gluten free and glutened foods, she baked the gluten free bread alongside the wheat bread in the oven, and she didn't wash her fingers when she went from handling foods with wheat, to those that didn't. Moreover, she didn't know what types of gluten free products to buy, so she didn't purchase the better tasting products. Plus, she didn't cook the gluten free products in the best way possible because she was unfamiliar with them, and she was in too much of a hurry to make them well. She tried, but good intentions aren't enough to ensure a satisfactory, safe, dining experience for people with gluten sensitivity.

Hooray for the hostess who tries to have gluten free foods available and proactively anticipates her guests' dietary needs. The issue of cross contamination is an innocent one for normal people who are cooking at home. The best thing the hostess can do is to anticipate potential problems and avoid them. Using clean pans and not re-using cutting boards or utensils is a good starting point. Making people aware she tried is at least emotionally comforting to the gluten free visitor. Being open to questions is important, because then the guests and hostess can have a fair and informative exchange about food issues. If the hostess is trying hard to do the right thing, she may be reluctant to disclose potential contamination that may have occurred. This puts the responsibility on the guest to ask questions and figure out which foods are safe and which are not. We always hope the hostess will gracefully accept such inquiries gracefully; getting defensive is an unfortunate outcome.

When a hostess invites folks to dinner and is the sole cook and bottle-washer, then the entire responsibility for a successful dining experience lies on her shoulders. This means planning ahead and being attentive to detail. It's useful to cook foods ahead of time so they can be safely and appropriately prepared, and then heated at the last minute. This helps reduce contamination through the hustle and bustle that often occurs when a hostess is trying to do too many things at the same time—and present a fabulous image.

We have no problem with a hostess making a public announcement before eating that some people (you don't have to say who) have gluten allergies, so everyone should be attentive to this issue. Especially if people are drinking alcohol, they may forget to be careful when taking food.

Attentive hosts create grateful guests, and possibly an invitation to their home—where they will likely create a lovely experience and be attentive to your dining needs as well.

Pot luck dinners

Churches, schools, clubs, families, and other groups love to hold pot luck dinners where everyone brings a favorite dish to share with others. The problem is, you don't know what your food options will be until you get there, and you don't know what's hidden in the dishes. You always have the option of bringing your own gluten free food and serving yourself first, but that takes all the fun out of pot luck.

Here are suggestions for a more successful, and healthy, pot luck experience for people who have gluten sensitivities:

Encourage everyone to be attentive to food allergies and bring the recipe, complete with a list of ingredients, to put alongside their dish. This way, everyone knows what's in it, and if they like the food, they can copy the recipe without bothering the person who brought the dish.

If you have gluten sensitivity, of course you'll bring a dish you like and can safely eat, but you must be the first to try it, in order to avoid contamination. The earlier you can serve yourself, the less risk there will be of someone creating a problem for you. You may feel rude by going first, since conventional manners encourage people to wait for others, but when it comes to not getting glutened, you need to put your health first. Everyone should understand and be supportive of this decision.

Hospital food

One would expect that a hospital, of all places, would have good, healthy food people with celiac disease can eat. We've found that isn't always the case. Early on, the hospital staff should note your dietary restrictions. When Chris was hospitalized once, he was served pre-packaged gluten free bread. That clearly meant it hadn't been exposed to any cross-contamination. His meal menus were specific for someone with a GF diet. This was super.

Unfortunately, all hospital dietary departments are not created equal. Once, Chris developed intense stomach pain with bleeding, which called for a trip to the local hospital. Several hospital clinics in the United States focus on the diagnosis and treatment of celiac disease, and we're fortunate enough to live near one of them. The medical team gave him an early appointment. He fasted and followed their instructions preparing for a colonoscopy, and arrived at the hospital where he underwent this procedure. When he awakened in the recovery room, a friendly nurse was there to give him juice and a snack so he could get his sugar levels up and help his stomach to start moving again. What snack was offered at the clinic? Graham crackers. Graham is not appropriate for someone who is gluten intolerant. He passed on the offer, and the hospital staff apologized, realizing it was a totally unacceptable food to offer someone with celiac disease. They assured him they would stock up on gluten free crackers. Six months later when he had a re-check, the same thing happened. Even though the staff recognized the need for gluten free snacks, none were available. They didn't run out of them—they never had them on hand to begin with.

Health care professionals are supposed to be attentive to basic needs like not giving a patient food that will make him sick. The wrong food can trigger problems with a variety of health conditions; sugar, salt, lactose, and gluten are the most common danger foods.

We recommend carrying your own snacks, just to be safe.

Amusement and sports park dining

Going to a ball game with the family is fun, and though the tickets are pricey, the entertainment and family time is worth the cost. Most sports facilities don't allow fans to bring their own food, because they hope each patron will buy a drink and a snack. We love going to Fenway Park to watch the Boston Red Sox and have found over the years they've become more sensitive to the needs of gluten free customers. They have a special gluten free stand where Chris can get a Fenway Frank on the bun with the safe Heinz and French's condiments, safe caramel corn, and ice cream. However, not all sports facilities are like this. You'd be advised to check the menu options in advance by calling the park. Some will have many options, while others have none. Don't assume there will be safe food.

Amusement parks are another family treat—and sooner or later you'll want something to eat. At a carry-in park, it's easy to pack a cooler full of food everyone can enjoy. Parks that forbid this practice make it hard for folks who have to go gluten free, unless the park offers special options. One park we like has a no carry-in-food policy, but we can usually find something safe to eat if we're not picky. On one particular day, that wasn't the case. The park purchased food from a single food distributor who did not provide gluten free options. Even the potentially safe food was prepared on contaminated surfaces. We watched as we ordered a cheeseburger sandwich without the bun— and realized the server had never changed gloves after plunking a hot dog into a bun. When we asked the server to make another cheese-between-lettuce leaves "sandwich" for us, he copped a big attitude, and made the food on a surface that had bread crumbs on it. When we requested yet another sandwich and tried to instruct the server about why we couldn't eat it, the lengthening line of annoyed people behind us caused us to leave without getting anything to eat.

Amusement parks usually don't have the physical space to prepare complicated food items, or the time to do so. An irregular request can create havoc for them, especially when impatient customers are lined up. Since the people working the food booths may not be trained about the gluten issue, we understand why they become frustrated. But why not have pre-packaged gluten free foods available? Simple food, such as fresh fruit or packaged carrots, would interest a variety of consumers, not just those who are gluten free. If a vendor knew even one place in the park where gluten free food was available, that information could be shared with the customer. Being curt to people trying to buy gluten free is a turn-off for everyone.

Business Meetings

Now that I understand the importance of having safe food for people with food allergies, we are much more sensitive to the needs of others. I think about all the meetings we've attended where they offered nothing we could eat. For instance, Chris was a guest speaker somewhere and his hosts nicely provided a pizza dinner, without realizing there was no way he could eat it. We've gone to business luncheons and realized too late here was nothing safe for him to consume.

I recently hosted a business open house and chose to serve cheese and crackers. But the cheese cubes were on a separate plate with toothpicks for removing them. This kept people from touching them with potentially contaminated hands. Crackers were on another plate. A box of gluten free crackers sat between them, so there was no chance of cross contamination. I did the same thing with cookies: Wheat based cookies were on a plate, far from the rest of the fruit I served, and I left a bag of gluten free cookies beside it. After the event was over, I realized people had gratefully consumed all the gluten free foods. Some took the GF foods with gratitude for actually being able to eat at the meeting. Others surely nibbled at them out of curiosity to see what gluten free food tasted like. Many people came back for seconds. The way we presented the food made it clear that gluten free is normal. There was no chance for contamination, and everyone could eat together in a spirit of community. This took little cost or effort on my part—just a little sensitivity and planning.

Summary

The issue of gluten free food touches every aspect of our dining experiences. As the case studies illustrate, people in charge of preparing food for others have many options for serving gluten free items. They can do so with upfront and clear information, or they can be intentionally or accidently deceptive. They can make sure the preparation is safe, or they can risk contamination. They can make delicious meals, or fix foods that people prefer not to eat. Guests can feel cared for and respected as they dine, or feel as though their needs don't matter. Eating, as we must always remember, is not just a nutritional experience. It is a social one as well.

When you go out to eat, your job is to become an advocate for yourself and make sure you eat safely. Take nothing for granted. Be willing to ask questions and tell people what you need. Others can't read your mind or decipher hints. You are NOT being annoying by making sure your food issues are addressed.

Everyone can go out to eat and have a safe, delicious experience. More and more people who deal with food are figuring out how to do GF well. But until you know for sure, protect yourself and educate the people around you. Guess who else benefits? The next person who needs to eat gluten free.

Chapter 6
How to Cook Gluten Free

Gluten free Foods Are Delicious. Surprised?

IF YOU ARE, that's probably because you've tried the wrong products or foods that weren't properly cooked. At first, gluten free cooking seemed hard to us and the available products were so awful that going gluten free felt like facing life-imprisonment. Now, we are gourmet gluten free cooks, and people scramble to dine with us because they know they're guaranteed to have a lovely meal.

Many books and websites now offer gluten free recipes. Even some mainstream cookbooks contain chapters for people with gluten intolerance or celiac disease, so there's no reason for you to spend lots of money on a gluten free cooking program. The gluten free community has done an excellent of providing information and recipes online—these folks know how hard it is to eat safely and they want to help. When people find good products and recipes, they love sharing them with others.

There are too many free GF recipe websites to list, but here are a few you may want to review:

All Recipes.com: http://bit.ly/1I204a0

Celiac.com: http://bit.ly/1CupB7e

Gluten free Goddess: http://glutenfreegoddess.blogspot.com/

Gluten free Works: http://glutenfreeworks.com/

King Arthur Flour: www.kingarthurflour.com/recipes

National Foundation for Celiac Awareness: http://bit.ly/1NBbiAG

Recipe Finders: http://bit.ly/1xwVVHl

Wheat free: http://bit.ly/1C4gbvo

Our Gluten Free Cooking Approach

I come from a family of good cooks. My mom and her sisters were country girls who grew up on a farm and learned how to grow their own foods and cook them into delicious dishes. Long before the terms became fashionable, they were organic, green, and sustainable. My mama baked her own breads, cakes, and cookies from scratch, as she called it. While we certainly had our share of processed foods and dining out experiences, the focus was always clear—you got the best food by growing it yourself and cooking at home. Simple food was best, but simple foods could be made to be delicious and even elegant. We used a basic recipe for most foods that could be adjusted, tweaked, and modified to turn into a wide array of amazing dishes. This was the food rendition of the little black dress—you could dress it up, down, and transform one basic item into a hundred different food experiences.

The critical factor in my cooking education was mastering the basic recipes and how to modify them, which made us into cooking chemists. We were kitchen scientists. We learned through trial and error; dishes that worked well we made again; ingredients that didn't turn out good food were modified or dropped from our repertoire. We were willing to make mistakes and take risks.

The thought of exact measuring was unfamiliar. I learned to develop a relationship with my food as we cooked. Kneading bread "until it's soft as a baby's butt" was the measure of when it was kneaded enough; instructions like "knead for ten minutes" never made sense to me. Recipes that called for a certain amount of an ingredient were ripe for modification. After all, the amounts were merely guidelines, not mandates. For instance, I like to use black pepper in dishes and if a recipe calls for 1/4 teaspoon, I may disregard that and use closer to 2 teaspoons, depending on the taste I want and who I'm cooking for. For major items, such as flour, sugar, or butter, I would stick closer to the recipe because they were the base. Of course I couldn't say exactly how much water to add because I never measured the flour and sugar exactly anyway. I learned to cook by knowing when something looked right. Many ingredients had amounts that were up for grabs. This is how I developed my imagination, creativity, and culinary courage.

This approach to cooking made my transference into gluten free cooking easier. Looking at the regular recipe and knowing it could be adapted freed me to adapt the base as well as additional ingredients. If a recipe called for flour, I knew I couldn't use wheat, so what other flours could I use? I found a large array of flours out there, none of which I'd known about except for rice flour. Rice may be fine for some products, but when I make pecan bars, coconut flour is much more delightful than wheat flour ever was in the recipe. When I make cream of potato soup, what type of flour is best? Why, potato flour, of course! If I want flour that will thicken well, tapioca flour is a good choice. **I recommend any gluten free cook get to know different flours. Play with them and experiment.**

Through this willingness to take risks and logically transform recipes, I've been able to turn many of our favorite glutened recipes into delightful gluten free ones. Sometimes they're even better than the original wheat based food. Other times, they are tasty, interesting, and have merit on their own. Cooking is Zen—you should have a basic plan, use a recipe as a guide, but free yourself from expectations. Sometimes a dish doesn't turn out exactly the way you expected, but you may be surprised and pleased with what you create.

Yvonne M. Vissing, Ph.D.
Christopher Moore-Vissing, BA

The following pages contain my my unique cooking approach with a base for most foods and then my variations. Many of the following recipes are my own creations.

My cooking approach may not work well for those of you who need tight structure and clear guidelines. In the following recipes I try to give close estimates for the key ingredients, but feel free to tweak the instructions. If this model works for you, wonderful! If not, then you should buy a cookbook that has strict rules to follow.

Sample Recipes

Salads

Diversity Tossed Salad

Fresh, varied, and interesting is the way we like it! Imagine ordering a salad and getting a quarter-head of iceberg lettuce plunked down in front of you, garnished by a few shredded carrots and a limp slice of tomato. On the other hand, imagine a salad that reflects the diversity of vegetables. In this salad, we alter the ingredients to match what we have fresh in our garden, or whatever looks good in the store. Here are the staples:

The Base: Baby spinach, romaine lettuce, and spring greens are the base of the salad, but don't rely on this to be the biggest ingredient. Using plenty of other vegetables will make every bite an experience, each mouthful different than the bite before. One of the biggest failures in salad making is using too much of the base and being skimpy with other ingredients. That's why so many people dislike restaurant salads.

Essential Other Vegetables: Add liberal amounts of carrots, tomatoes, onions, cucumber, and peppers. You can vary the preparation. Carrots can be chunked, shredded, crinkled, or baby types; tomatoes may be big and beefy, cherry, grape, or plum—they may also be red, yellow or green. Peppers can be yellow, orange, purple, red, dark green, light green, or any size, from short and fat to long and thin, to sweet to very, very hot. Onions can be purple or yellow, shallots, chives, or little and green. Cukes may be European and elegant or the bumpy grown-in-your-garden pickling type. These choices will make the salad look and taste different every time.

Optional Veggies: We love radishes, celery, sprouts, broccoli, cauliflower, and fresh mushrooms, but not everyone agrees. Avocado, beets and asparagus are other vegetables that may be questionable; while we like them, not everyone does. We are sensitive to the palate of our guests and modify the salad ingredients to please them.

Don't Forget the Uncommon: Leafy vegetables like kale, arugula, cabbage, chicory, watercress can make a salad interesting. Likewise, using fresh basil, cilantro, parsley and other herbs create tastes that give each salad a different flavor. Do you like roasted red peppers? Artichoke hearts? Anything can go in a salad. Jalapenos, peppers, and other vegetables in brine add zing to a salad and make other dressing unnecessary. Banana pepper slices tossed into a salad can be delightful—but only if you like that kind of spiciness.

Olives: (green or black), pitted, unpitted, or stuffed, your choice! Olive varieties are endless.

Cheeses: We love fresh fontina or parmesan, but cheddar or provolone is also wonderful. Feta is necessary when transforming this dish into a Greek salad. Some people like blue cheese or gorgonzola. Buffalo mozzarella provides a heavenly Italian spin when served with tomatoes, black pepper, and fresh basil. In general, don't smother your fresh veggies with cheese. A little cheese enhances a salad; too much drowns it.

Beans, Peanuts, or Other Legumes: raw, soaked, salted, or vinegared, beans are another personal preference. Corn is another item to consider. If you're making a Mexican salad, kidney, or black beans and corn may work well; on a Cobb salad, perhaps not.

Meat, Fish and Eggs: People tend to either love eggs or hate them, and given today's vegan and cholesterol concerned guests, we tend not to put them on—but you could. If the salad is a main dish, then adding chicken, bacon, or other meats or fish may be desirable, but adding these is something that must be negotiated, not assumed.

Nuts: Almonds, walnuts, cashews, or pecans are our favorites. Sometimes we add coconut if we're going with a summer theme that includes slices of fruit, such as oranges or strawberries on the salad. Nuts can be raw, toasted, salted, glazed with sugar, or made spicy. The choice is yours, and each will take your salad in a different direction. But be careful—nut allergies abound and you can ruin someone's dinner, and health, by automatically adding nuts.

Fruits: Commonly used fruits include pineapple, oranges, strawberries, apples, grapes, and blueberries. Fruit salads require a carefully selected dressing, such as poppy seed, to make them work well.

Croutons: Yes, the delicious gluten free ones. See my recipe for them.

Grains: We usually don't add pasta, rice, or other carbohydrates to a fresh salad. Somehow, that seems to defeat our purpose. We prefer to use them in main dishes instead. But one could add them. In general, if we want a pasta or rice salad, that's what we'll make.

Theme Salads: The secret is to combine flavors that go together. If I'm making a salad with an Italian theme, I use basil but don't use cilantro; if it's a Mexican or springtime salad, I will use cilantro but not the basil. Sometimes I'll make an all green salad using spinach, cucumbers, peppers, artichokes, celery, etc. – all different types of green tastes and consistencies, with a homemade buttermilk ranch dressing, or maybe a vinaigrette. Other times I want color and use everything in the rainbow. Some people think salads are boring, when nothing could be further from the truth. They are good for us and the variety ends only when our creative juices stop flowing.

Flexible Dressing

Just as the salad varies by what you put into it, so does our salad dressing. We'll give you the base recipe, and then suggest ways to alter it for scrumptious salad dressings that will convince you never to buy the bottled kind again.

Base Dressing: In a blender or food processor, mix olive oil, then a choice of lemon/lime juice or apple cider/balsamic vinegar. Some people like the citrus acid and prefer lemon or lime juice, which gives the dressing a tart zing. Other people prefer vinegar. In general, we stay away from white vinegar, as it is questionable. Apple cider vinegar is always acceptable for gluten free menus. If you like a darker, heavier taste, use balsamic vinegar instead. With this base, you can have four different flavors, depending on what type of juice or vinegar you use.

Option 1: Vinaigrette dressing

If you want a vinegrette dressing, add the type of herbs you like. I like pepper a lot, and basil is another favorite. Add rosemary, thyme, parsley, garlic, dried onion, salt, or tarragon. Of course, if you have other favorites, add them to fit the menu you're serving.

Option 2: Vegetable dressing

This is a heavy, rich, and flavorful dressing that can even be used as a dip. Cut small pieces of the vegetables of your choice: Cucumbers, onions and celery are staples. If you want a more "green" type dressing, add green peppers and more of the above ingredients. Parsley is a good neutral herb. If you want more of an Italian flare, add basil; if you want more of a Middle Eastern or Mexican flavor, then add cilantro leaves. On the other hand, if you want a French type dressing, then add the red vegetables, such as tomatoes, red peppers, and carrots. Be careful to cut the peppers and carrots into small pieces before blending; it helps the process. The color and flavor of your dressing will depend upon what you choose.

Now comes the issue of spice. Some people like a neutral flavored dressing; others like a rosemary and tarragon taste, while still others want to add hot peppers, chili powder, cumin or coriander. You can add Boars Head, French's mustard, or Heinz ketchup if you want a mustardy or French type dressing. The amount all depends upon how much oil and other ingredients you use.

A cook has to deal with the texture concern; some people love thick dressings that are almost the consistency of dip, while others like them thin and fluid. This influences the decision of how much oil and vinegar/juice to add.

My personal favorite is to throw some tomatoes, cucumbers, onion, celery, peppers, olive oil, lime juice, cilantro, and chili powder into the blender. It comes out thick, red, spicy, and so good I love to eat it as a vegetable dip as well as a salad dressing. It must be other people's favorite too, because there's never any left.

Cooking is like chemistry—a process of trial and error to see what combinations work best for what purposes. There is seldom a right or wrong; how can you go wrong by mixing lovely vegetables together in various combinations? Think about what you have in the kitchen and how you want the end product to taste and appear—and then bravely experiment with new things. Take risks. Your confidence will increase, and your guests will be awed as you create a multitude of fresh, delicious sauces that are cheaper, healthier, and safer than store-bought dressings.

Croutons

Many gluten free people miss the simple things like croutons on salads. To buy them can be pricey, but it's a snap to make them with leftover bread. Use slices of gluten free bread, like Udi's, and cut them into squares. Sprinkle with olive oil, salt, pepper, or Parmesan cheese and put them into the oven to toast at 350 degrees until they're golden brown and crispy. These are delicious on salads, soups, or anything else that inspires you. They are so good that you'll never buy store croutons again, and you'll have an easy way to use stale bread.

Yvonne M. Vissing, Ph.D.
Christopher Moore-Vissing, BA

Enlightened Slaw

Growing up, I thought cole slaw always consisted of grated cabbage with Miracle Whip. It was heavy, goopey, homogenous white in color, but admittedly pretty darn tasty, especially on a ruben sandwich or with an order of fish-and-chips. But now I know a good cole slaw is a fine dish, even a delicacy, depending on how you make it. Here are some options:

The Base: The type of slaw you make depends upon the kind of cabbage you start with. There are the traditional green and purple varieties, but there are also Chinese cabbage (aka bok choy), savoy cabbage, and my new favorite, nappa cabbage. Some people like to use finely sliced broccoli instead of cabbage, as these vegetables are in the same family.

You can go to great effort to chop or grate cabbage, or buy it pre-grated. This decision depends on your preference. Home grated has an advantage because you can adjust. Next, add other vegetables of your choosing. Carrots, onion, celery and green/red pepper are typical choices, although some people just want cabbage and nothing else. Lately I've been adding lots of little radish pieces, cucumber, and cilantro. Personally, I love color and like to tie the themes together. Food should look as good as it tastes, and should be a feast for the eyes as well as the palate. The more other vegetables you add, the less cabbage you have, which gives an entirely different taste and presentation.

Now comes the critical decision: how do you want to bind the slaw together? Sometimes a lime juice or vinegar and sugar theme is desired; it makes for a sweet and sour slaw that's light to the taste. Often I will add celery seed to this, mix it well, and let it sit for a while so the flavors have a chance to mingle and blend. I find this works well in the summer and keeps freshness high.

On the other hand, you may like a combination of vinegar and mayo, which is a favorite type. The mayo will bind it together, while the vinegar adds pizzazz. If you do this, don't use too much mayo or you'll end up with a sloppy mess. You don't want to hide the crispness of the vegetables in the mayo, but rather allow them to cling together and keep their independence.

For a mayonnaise base, you have several choices that include real mayonnaise, a gluten free product like Miracle Whip, or making your own mayo.

Here is my homemade mayonnaise recipe if you want to try it instead of using a commercial product. It is different from what you may be used to, but very lovely.

Homemade Mayonnaise

1 cup of light olive oil (I like this much better than the virgin, which I find to have a harsh taste)

Juice from 1 lemon, lemon juice, or cider vinegar – how much actually depends upon how zingy you like your dressing.

1 egg

salt

pepper

Directions: Add egg and vinegar/juice and mix well. Then pour in the olive oil slowly, a little at a time, beating regularly with a blender, food processor, or by hand if you're diligent. It should thicken up. If the mixture is too thick, you can add a little water or vinegar. When you have the texture you want, add salt and pepper (or mustard, dill seed, celery seed, or other flavors) to taste. That's all there is to it. You can mix it with your hands for best results. Taste frequently and doctor it until you reach perfection.

Yvonne M. Vissing, Ph.D.
Christopher Moore-Vissing, BA

Soups

Soup is the easiest thing in the world to make. Remember the childhood story of Stone Soup? If you have a pan, water, and something edible to put in it, you can make soup. You don't even need to add a rock. Usually, soup is never made exactly the same way twice, so liberate yourself from the idea of a recipe. Be creative, daring, and brave. I'm giving you the quick, easy, basic recipes, and over time, you will become more sophisticated and make variations. Usually soup doesn't cost much to make, so if you make a batch you don't like, simply throw it away and try again. The more you make soup, the better you'll become as a gourmet soup chef.

Here are basic soup categories:

Vegetable soup

Legume soup

Cream soup

Cold soup

and then, there's Chili!

Vegetable Soups

Basic soup base

Every soup needs a base to build on. I use gluten free chicken stock. If you buy it, read the ingredients to determine if yours is gluten free or not. If you're a vegetarian, buy veggie broth or use broth left over from cooking other vegetables, such as potato broth left over from mashing them or making potato salad. That leftover broth is nutritious, and it's a shame to dump it down the sink. If you stick it in the refrigerator in a pitcher, you can simply pour it into your pan to make soup another day. But don't keep it more than three days—the rule is, you can eat leftovers for three days, but the fourth day they should be thrown out. Once you have a soup base, all you need to do is mix other ingredients to create the type you want.

Fundamental Vegetable Soup

My favorite vegetable soup is simple and contains only five vegetables and seasoning. In a pot, put a can of tomatoes (I like the pureed or diced kind—the whole tomatoes are just too big unless you cut them into pieces) and add broth. As this begins to boil, add fresh carrot hunks, potato chunks, celery slices, and a small diced onion. Throw it all together, add black pepper, salt and a bay leaf or two if you have them, and yummmm! This is soup most people rave about the most. Simple is best. (PS – never eat the bay leaves; it is best to remove them before serving).

Veggie Soup Variations

Stew: If you cut the potato, celery, and carrot pieces bigger and use less liquid and cook it low and slow so it thickens up, you'll have stew. You may add beef, chicken pieces, or even tofu to create a stew with protein.

Pasta or Rice: Toss in a handful of rice or pasta to make the soup heartier. Don't use both at the same time—one or the other, and maybe neither, if you're using many potato or root vegetables in your soup. Too much carbohydrate loading leads to soup that resembles paste when you reheat it tomorrow. If you use gluten free pasta, cook it separately and add just a little before serving. While rice can be cooked in the vegetable broth, gluten free pasta has a way of dissolving when cooked too long.

Other Vegetables: You can add almost any vegetables to your soup. In some ways, the more the merrier. Having cabbage, broccoli, asparagus, beans, zucchini, little pieces of squash, etc., turns your simple soup into Garden Vegetable. However, I usually avoid green peppers and mushrooms in my soup, as they tend to get slimy.

Quickie Vegetable Soup: Soup need not take a huge amount of time or complications. Put broth in pan, add two plus cans of mixed vegetables, a can of tomatoes, a can of beans, and some rice or pasta, salt and pepper, In 15 minutes it's done.

Leftovers Soup: Whatever leftover vegetable, rice or meat you have in the fridge can easily be turned into soup. I'll often look and see I have a little bowl of this or that, and instead of tossing them out, I throw everything into a pot with broth and other vegetables, legumes, or grains to turn it into soup. Leftover Mexican beans and rice can become tortilla soup; leftover Italian can become Minestrone, leftover Indian dishes can become awesome curry soup. Sometimes this technique of making soup results in an odd dish, but usually they're surprisingly wonderful. Take a risk instead of wasting food. Give it a fun name. Maybe this new soup will be so popular you'll transform it into a menu staple.

Minestrone Soup. Use the basic recipe (tomatoes, potatoes, onion, celery and carrots), and add a handful of pasta and a can of red kidney beans. Some folks like to add squash (yellow or zucchini) or red/green peppers. Season it black pepper, lots of basil, and a bay leaf. When the vegetables and pasta are soft—it's done! Serve with parmesan cheese on top.

Mulligatawny Soup: Use the above recipe for Minestrone soup, only season it with curry powder or cumin and coriander instead of the basil. You can substitute garbanzo or white beans for the red beans to give it more of that Indian essence.

Winter Vegetable Soup. Use the basic broth, then onion and cooked butternut squash. You can also add potatoes, parsnips, turnips, or carrots. This is a savory soup, so put in a bay leaf, thyme, rosemary and savory, along with salt and pepper to taste.

Ki's Onion Soup

This is a gluten free variation of a long standing favorite.

1 quart chicken soup broth	4 large Spanish onions
5 ounces butter	2 cups water
1 bay leaf	1/4 teaspoon thyme
1 teaspoon lemon juice	Salt and pepper

Sliced gluten free bread; I often turn mine into croutons
Grated Gruyere cheese (or Swiss)

Cut onions into quarters and slice them. Sauté the slices in butter until they are tender and golden. Pour them into broth with water, herbs, lemon juice, and brandy. Simmer for almost an hour. Pour soup into small bowls, top with gluten free bread or croutons and top it with cheese. Bake or broil them for a few minutes to let the cheese melt, and serve immediately. Yum!

Chicken Noodle or Chicken Rice Soup

I can think of many variations on these basic chicken soups, but here's a good place to start: Place chicken broth into a pan and do one of the following:

a) open a can of chicken and toss it in,

b) cut chicken breasts or strips into small pieces and toss them into the pot, or

c) cook the actual chicken in with the broth.

If you use a whole chicken, you'll have to deal with the skin and bones later, which I find time consuming and messy. That's why I use boneless breasts if possible. Once you've established your chicken base, add a little celery, carrots, black pepper, and decide if you want to add gluten free noodles or rice. Be careful not to add too much of the rice or noodles—both tend to swell and you'll be amazed at how thick it gets, which makes it hard to enjoy that good chicken broth.

Legume Soups

Bean, lentil, and pea soups are hearty, delicious, and nutritious. But cooking with legumes can be a challenge because they stay hard unless cooked long enough. That's why some people resort to using canned legumes. The canned varieties make great soup and are much faster. However, you'll probably want to develop your cooking skills with dry legumes.

You'll also find that legume-based soups often taste better on the second day. The first day they're on the thin side, but letting them sit in the fridge and serving them the next day gives you a thicker, tastier soup. In other words, these soups get better with age. Here's the scoop about particular kinds of legumes:

Lentils, split green peas, and split yellow peas cook fastest, while black beans, kidney beans, navy beans, and whole pea beans (white or colored) take longer. Some people let them sit overnight in water to soak and soften. If you do let the legumes soak, drain off the old water and use fresh water for cooking. Sometimes when I'm in a hurry, I'll boil water and then add the beans, which makes them cook faster. If you use a pressure cooker, they actually cook fast.

Shuggie's Lentil Soup

Put lentils into broth and add crushed tomatoes as a base, then add vegetables. When I'm in a hurry I use a can or two of mixed vegetables (or frozen), but I recommend fresh vegetables like carrots, onions, and celery. I don't use potatoes since that makes for too much carbohydrate, in my opinion. The ratio of lentils to water tells you how thick the soup will be—and that's a bigger issue on the second day, so think ahead. Many people like their soup thick with chunky carrots and celery pieces, and they call it lentil stew.

Split Pea Soup

Put peas into broth, then add onions, and bacon, ham, or hickory seasoning for vegetarians. Gluten free smoky seasoning is excellent. Cook until soft and eat.

My Curried Dal Soup

Yellow spit peas are the basis for dal. Put the yellow peas into water or broth with curry seasonings, especially cumin and coriander. Add vegetables (fresh, canned or frozen). I am partial to carrots, onion and celery. Let the soup cook until soft and thick. Pea soup is wonderful, especially in the winter when served with bread and salad.

Bean Soup

Bean soups, like vegetable soups, vary with what you put into them. You can use only one type of bean or a combination. Some people gather every kind of bean or legume they can find, throw them in together, and make a mixed bean soup that can be a knock-out. Similarly, you can skip the vegetables and add only onion, or go with onion, celery and carrots. I usually don't add any other vegetables to bean soup besides those three. You can use a chicken broth base or add fresh or canned tomatoes for a tomato base. Sometimes I'll add some hickory smoke and a bay leaf too, but these aren't essential. Remember, the trick with bean soup is plan ahead and give it plenty of time to cook. I don't know how beans cook in the microwave, but I imagine it could be done, especially if you add plenty of water in a lidded glass dish.

A Version of Spicy Lentil and Tomato Soup
Chris learned about in Oxford

When Chris was studying in Oxford, England, he discovered this wonderful variation of lentil soup.

1 medium onion	1 clove garlic
1 teaspoon coriander	1 teaspoon turmeric
2 teaspoons chili powder	1 can green lentils or 1 cup dried lentils
1 can chopped tomatoes	2 pints vegetable or chicken stock

Cream Soups

Cream soups are something many gluten free people miss because cooks don't know how to adjust recipes for them. In general, cream soups take a smidge longer to make, but I think they're a nicer, more elegant soup and preparing them gluten free takes no more time than making them with wheat flour. Cream soups are especially good when it's cold as a comfort food. Like the other soups, start with a basic cream soup recipe and then add variations.

Basic Cream Soup and Variations

Melt two Tablespoons of butter in a pan. Then mix in a couple Tablespoons of gluten free flour. My favorite is King Arthur Gluten Free Flour because it is light and the texture is similar to wheat flour. Mixing the flour and butter creates a yellow, goopy paste. Work fast so it doesn't stick. Then slowly add about two cups of milk. This thickens the paste and if you use a whisk it won't become lumpy. Whisks are useful for making cream soups, but not essential. Just be prepared to break up the lumps so you don't eat a mouthful of clumped flour.

Season this mixture with salt, pepper, parsley, or a bay leaf if you want. A little dried parsley makes the cream soups look pretty. Once you have the cream base, add the other ingredients. For instance, if you want a very creamy soup, add more milk. If you want a thinner cream soup, add chicken or vegetable broth.

The secret to making a decent cream soup is cooking your vegetables in water in a separate pan, and then adding them to the base. If you're making potato soup, put the potato and carrot and celery and onion pieces in a pan with water (plus seasonings if you want), and when they're soft, add them to the cream base. Same thing with carrot soup (usually it's good to smush the carrots so it's all pretty instead of lumpy). Use the same technique for zucchini, asparagus, cauliflower, or broccoli. When you mix the two pans of ingredients together, you may decide you'd like a thicker soup. If that's the case, I recommend you scoop out a little hot broth, add the gluten free flour to it, get it smooth, then pour it into the pan. If you add flour directly to the broth in the pot, you'll get clumps, or "dumplings." I've been known to scoop out big clumps with a serving spoon before dinner, just because it's hard to get rid of all the lumps.

You can add cheese to the cream soup to make cheddar potato, cheddar cauliflower, or cheddar broccoli soups. I like the cheesy soup, and feel it provides extra protein. Adding bread or crackers gives you a great meal.

If you want to make cream of tomato, create the flour/butter/milk base, cook the tomatoes and whatever else separately, and then put everything together. You can also cook rice separately and throw it into tomato soup, which makes it wonderful. Not too much rice, though, because it swells with time and you'll find two days later that all you have is seasoned rice, not soup. The only time I use leeks is in a potato leek soup. Leeks are a sort of onion so a few are okay, but too many leeks will overwhelm the other ingredients.

Some good cream soup combinations are:

Potatoes	Broccoli
Cauliflower	Asparagus
Carrots (or carrot-ginger)	Cheese soup

Pumpkin Squash Soup

3 cans pumpkin	1 small diced onion
1 medium squash, cubed	3 cups chicken broth
1 teaspoon butter	1 teaspoon gluten free flour
2 Tablespoon brown sugar	1 cup cream
Salt, pepper, ginger, cinnamon to taste	

Saute the onions and squash in butter. Mash when it is soft. Add to the chicken broth and simmer. Stir in pumpkin. Mix flour, butter, sugar, and spices. Fold in cream last. Heat but do not boil.

Cheesy Cauliflower Soup

5 Tablespoons butter

1 head of cauliflower, chopped

1 teaspoon parsley

3 Tablespoon GF flour

1 cup cheddar and parmesan cheeses

1 onion

6 cups chicken stock

1 teaspoon dill

Cream of Potato Carrot Soup

3 Tablespoons butter

1/2 to 1 lb carrots

2 Tablespoon dill

6 cups chicken stock

1 onion

4 potatoes

1 teaspoon sage

1 cup half and half or cream

Cream of Butternut Squash

2 butternut squash, peeled and cubed

1 Tablespoon cinnamon

8 cups chicken broth

1/2 pint half and half or cream

1 Tablespoon nutmeg

Cream of Ginger Carrot Soup

Melt 5 Tablespoons butter and sauté 1 lb carrots, 1 onion, 1 lb ginger, and add to 3 cups chicken stock, 2 cups cream, marjoram, salt and pepper. Ginger has a quirky taste that people tend to love or hate.

Chowders

Chowders are a New England specialty and fall into three common types—corn chowder, fish chowder, or seafood chowder.

The Base: All chowders start with a thin cream soup base that has extra cream or half-and-half in addition to milk, plus a good dose of butter. Having the yellow butter residue float on top is classic.

Corn Chowder: This is nothing more than chunky cream of corn and potato soup with a bit of onion added. (I add celery and carrots because I like them. I don't guess they're actually necessary to make corn chowder, but it sounds more elegant, doesn't it?) Just cut the potatoes in hunks, add the butter, and that's chowder.

Sometimes people transform corn chowder into Mexi corn chowder by eliminating the potatoes and adding cilantro, cumin, coriander, green chilies, and some tomatoes to the mix. This gives it an entirely different taste and appearance. It can be made as spicy as you like by varying the amount of chilies and spices.

Fish Chowder: Use the base (cream, butter, milk, potatoes, salt and pepper) with hunks of fish that cook in the broth. Use haddock, cod, or some other mild fish. Fishy tasting fish isn't appetizing.

Seafood Chowder: This the same as fish chowder, but substitute shrimp, scallops, or whatever other "food from the sea" you want.

Cold Soups

Cold soups can be vegetable or fruit based. They're actually easy, but you usually need a blender or food processor.

Cold Potato Soup (vischoisse)

Make regular cream of potato soup and garnish with scallions or leeks. Chill it, and you have an an elegant summer soup. If you need a recipe, try this one:

2 Tablespoon butter	1 onion, chopped
4 potatoes	4 leeks, white part only

1/2 cup chopped dill

3 cups chicken stock

1-1/2 cups cream

1-1/2 cups milk

Cold Blueberry Soup

5 cups or 2 lb. crushed frozen blueberries

3 cups orange juice

I can of frozen orange juice

1/2 cup sugar

4 cups vanilla yogurt

1 cup sour cream

orange peel

Fresh mint leaves for garnish

dash of cinnamon, grated

Blend together all ingredients and serve cold.

Thanks to Walter Baily of Maine for this yummy recipe!

Cold Strawberry Soup

4 cup strawberries, crushed

1/4 cup sugar

1 teaspoon cinnamon

4 cups vanilla yogurt

Strawberry halves for garnish

Blend together all ingredients and serve cold

Gazpacho

Everyone seems to have their own preference for this soup. You can make it redder by using lots of tomatoes/tomato juice, or more green by using lots of cucumbers and celery. You can make it as spicy as you want, or not spicy at all. Here are the most typical ingredients, but you don't need to use all of them. Put whatever you like into the food processor/blender, and then spice it to suit your palate, chill, and enjoy!

Essential ingredients: Tomatoes, cucumbers, celery, onion, lemon juice or cider vinegar, olive oil.

Optional: Spicy V-8 Juice, tomato juice, green pepper, cilantro, parsley

Spices to choose from: Tabasco, salsa, cumin, coriander, chili powder, jalapenos

Other Fruit Soups

Think of using any fruit you have around, mixing it with fruit juice you already have, and any yogurt available. Voila—fruit soup! Thicker, it could be a smoothie. Thin it until you have a soup consistency. These soups are easy to make and delicious on a hot day. Raspberries, strawberries, and peaches, mixed with orange or apple juice and yogurt are wonderful. Make it elegant by adding a few fresh berries or something else to garnish the top.

Chilli

Chili is practically the national soup of the United States, with regional favorites and cook-offs across the country. Be a scientist and create your own chili, based on the recipe my grandma always used:

Onion, chopped	Ground beef or turkey
Tomatoes (canned)	Spaghetti or other pasta
Beans (canned red beans are good)	
Chili powder and other spices	
Cheese to sprinkle on top	

Boil the water, add cut up onion, tomatoes, beans, and chili powder to taste. Then add browned ground beef or turkey. Grandma always put in spaghetti—the thin kind , but many people don't use any pasta, or serve the bean/meat mixture over pasta. I recommend using corn based pasta, as it hangs together well. Rice pasta has a tendency to be slimy. Some people sprinkle cheese on top. You may add other spices to make it hot, or buy pre-made chili spice. Although your chili may be thin at first, the pasta swells and by day three it will be thick.

You can easily transform this chili into a vegetarian dish by skipping the meat and adding more beans and whole kernel corn, if you like. Some people like to add black, red, pink, white, or other types of beans. You can also toss in chili peppers.

Yvonne M. Vissing, Ph.D.
Christopher Moore-Vissing, BA

Main Dishes

Pasta

Pasta dishes are easy, quick, and cheap to make. They can even be elegant. You'll find dozens of pasta types to choose from, plus all kinds of sauces to mix and match.

You'll see long spaghettis, such as fettuccini (which is long and flat), angel hair (long and very skinny), and pericotelli, which is round, fat and long. Regular spaghetti and many other types are also long and thin. Shorter, fatter pastas are ziti, elbows, or rigatoni. Some pasta can be stuffed, such as big shells and lasagna noodles, whereas other shells make great dishes like macaroni and cheese. Risotto is a wonderful substitution for pasta: delicious, and gluten free.

Just because you can't eat wheat pasta doesn't mean you can't enjoy this delicious food. You'll be able to find a large variety of gluten free pastas. Some are made with rice, some with quinoa, and others are made from corn. Corn is my personal favorite, but many types are available, with new ones coming on the market every year.

Basic sauce categories include:

Bechamel sauce: This delicious sauce can be used for a zillion foods—as a base for macaroni and cheese, to top walnut cheese balls, as a cream soup base, over green vegetables like asparagus, or whatever you want. You can turn it into Alfredo sauce by adding Parmesan cheese. You can modify it easily to meet the needs of whatever you're making. This a super recipe I use often:

Ingredients:

1/2 onion	3 Tablespoons melted butter
3 Tablespoons gluten free four	Milk

Sauté the onion and add melted butter. Mix in 3 Tablespoon gluten free flour and add milk, keeping the mixture smooth, not lumpy. Add milk to reach the consistency you want. Add herbs.

This sauce keeps well, so make extra to keep for later.

Red sauces: Red sauce can be as simple as opening a can or bottle from the grocery, or you may choose to make your own sauce from scratch. A good homemade red sauce can take days to cook, starting thin and getting thick and rich as the days go by. My homemade red sauces tend to be fast—I sauté in olive oil fresh tomatoes, a little garlic, an onion, maybe some green peppers, and always LOTS of basil. It doesn't matter if the basil is fresh or dried—use a lot of it. Basil is the secret ingredient. You can add oregano or rosemary, or buy an Italian seasoning mix to add. But if you can only have one seasoning, use basil.

You can also purchase gluten free red sauce at the store and add basil, vegetables, or red wine to it to make a unique sauce that is fast, good, and cheap. Be careful about using premade pasta sauce, because many of these contain tomato paste thickened with a gluten product, which would make it unsafe. The more natural the product, the better.

Cheese sauces: Also called Alfredo sauces, these delectable sauces are easy to make. Basically, Alfredo sauce is a white sauce with lots of parmesan and Romano cheese. And for the white sauce, you'll create the same basic recipe you'd use to start a cream soup or a Bechemal sauce. All you do is melt butter, add gluten free flour, add milk and cream, salt, pepper, and cheeses. Simple, eh? Add as many different kinds of cheeses as you want to this sauce. But for macaroni and cheese, stick with sharp cheddar. It's the best.

Primavera sauces: Primavera is French for spring, color, and lots of vegetables cooked together in olive oil with basil to make a fresh sauce. No goopy red sauce here. Zucchini, tomatoes, peppers, onions, squash, pumpkin, eggplant—whatever you have on hand can turn into a delicious sauce. You decide how much of which vegetables. Just remember to cook them in olive oil and stir often.

Presto Pesto: Pesto sauce is easy to make, delicious, and more excellent homemade than you can imagine. The ingredients:

Light olive oil	Fresh basil
Black pepper	Parmesan cheese
Pine nuts	

You probably won't need to add salt, because the salt in the cheese should be enough. Pine nuts are expensive per pound, so the exact consistency of the pesto can be adjusted to meet your palate. You will need a blender or food processor to make pesto.

Take bunches of fresh basil, wash it, pick off the leaves, stuff the leaves into the processor. Add olive oil, and pine nuts. Grind together. Pour the mixture into a bowl and add parmesan cheese. Keep doing this until you get as much pesto as you want. I use at least a cup of leaves, a half cup or more of oil, and 2/3 cup or so of nuts. You may wish to add more or less oil until you get a spreadable consistency.

Serve this delicious sauce on warm pasta (it spreads easiest that way when you toss it), spread on gluten free bread along with some tomatoes and fresh mozzarella cheese to make a wonderful sandwich, or put it on top of polenta for an elegant and quick meal.

I love the cheese, so I add more than most people do. You can add a half cup of cheese while you blend, and then when you scoop it out, you add even more if you like. Enjoy!

Oil based sauces: Sometimes it's delicious to heat lots of olive oil in a skillet, add a pinch of garlic, and then add walnuts or pine nuts, along with tomatoes, artichoke hearts, and basil, then pour the resulting sauce over pasta. You can add fresh mozzarella cheese or sprinkle the regular kind of parmesan on top.

Nancy B's Sauce

Nancy is a fantastic cook and obtained this recipe from a girlfriend from South America.

2 cloves garlic, crushed

2 Tablespoon olive oil

3/4 red pepper cut in thin strips

2 large cans whole tomatoes

Stuffed Spanish olives sliced in good sized pieces

Black olives, if you want them

Fresh basil leaves

Saute the garlic and peppers in oil. Chop tomatoes and add (or buy crushed tomatoes and save yourself this cutting step). Add a hearty amount of basil (15 leaves+), salt and pepper to taste. You can add a little sugar if you want, since that's what the tomato sauce people do to make it extra-tasty. I like this recipe for a change of pace; the olives are great on pasta with cheese on top. I always add more basil because it's one of my favorite herbs.

Shuggie's Macaroni and Cheese

Melt butter in a pan, add gluten free flour, then add milk to make a pasty white sauce. Add seasonings like pepper, and cheddar cheese or whatever cheese you have around. Keep adding milk and cheese until you get the flavor and consistency you like. I like to use some parmesan too, because I think it gives you a nice salty taste. Muenster melts easily. You can make a quick mac and cheese on top the stove by cooking the pasta in one pan and the sauce in the other. Drain the pasta, and toss the sauce over the noodles. Voila! Dinner! Or, you can bake it by pouring the pasta-sauce mixture into a casserole, putting more cheese on top (or gluten free cracker crumbs), and bake in the oven. You'll need enough sauce to cover the pasta and be aware that it will dry a bit during baking. In other words—make more sauce than you think you'll need.

Yvonne M. Vissing, Ph.D.
Christopher Moore-Vissing, BA

Shuggie's Eggplant Parmesan

Eggplant, skinned and sliced thin

Seasonings (your choice)

Cracker or bread crumbs, gluten free

Olive oil

Beaten eggs and milk

Tomato sauce for topping

Cheese—mozzarella, provolone, or parmesan

Take the skin off an eggplant (or mini eggplants) with a vegetable scraper or knife. Cut the eggplant into very thin slices. If the pieces are too thick, it takes a long time for them to cook through, and they're not as tasty as thinly sliced pieces. Set the cut slices into bowl 1.

In bowl 2, put a mixture of gluten free cracker or bread crumbs. I like to add seasoning, such as pepper, basil, or (my favorite) Cajun seasoning. This yields a spicy, crispy coating that makes the eggplant marvelous!

In bowl 3, put milk, beaten eggs, or a mixture of both.

Heat a skillet with olive oil in it—and plan to use LOTS more olive oil than you think is healthy. The eggplant soaks it up like a sponge, and you will have to add more oil regularly to your skillet.

Now comes the fun. Dip an eggplant slice it into the milk/egg mixture, then dip it into the crumb mixture. Everything should hang together pretty well. Then put it into the oil to brown, flipping it over until both sides are golden brown. If the oil is too hot, the eggplant will burn. If you don't have enough batter on the eggplant, it isn't pretty. (I find I keep washing the crumb mixture off my fingers because it clumps after a while.)

Place the golden slices of breaded eggplant onto a plate and try to resist eating them. Once you start tasting, you'll never have enough. If the eggplant survives, put a layer of it in a pan covered with either tomato sauce or olive oil. Then top the eggplant with sauce and a thick covering of mozzarella, provolone, or parmesan cheese. Bake it. When it gets close to dinner time, boil water and make gluten free pasta so people can put the eggplant parmesan on top. Some people bake the entire eggplant mixture on top of the pasta, which is a beautiful presentation. Either way, it's wicked good. Enjoy.

Pizza Rustica

The original recipe for this pizza pie called for a wheat flour crust and top, just like a fruit pie. Gluten free pie crusts are challenging to make. Unless you find a product that meets your standards, I find it is easier to forgo the crusts and make a crustless variation. This dish ends up being delightful, even if it doesn't fit your traditional version of pizza.

Mix together:

5 eggs	3 fresh tomatoes
1 lb Ricotta cheese	2/3 cup olives (optional)
1/2 sauted onion	green pepper slices (optional)
1 Tablespoon garlic	1 cup mozzarella cheese
10 ounces tomato puree	1 cup Parmesan cheese
chopped parsley, basil, oregano, marjoram, salt, pepper	

Mix eggs, Ricotta, and Parmesan in a bowl together. Place a layer of it in the bottom of a pan oiled with olive oil. Then layer on the garlic, spices, and tomato mixture, which should be simmering on the stove. On top of the ricotta layer add the tomato layer, then a layer of mozzarella cheese, and do it all over again. Add peppers and olives in a layer if you want. Top with the tomato layer, then top with cheese. Bake at 375 for almost an hour. It is wonderful!

Lasagna Done Right

Lasagna is perhaps the easiest and most tasty of all gluten free Italian foods. Start with these ingredients:

Lasagna noodles, gluten free (made with rice, corn, or other flours)

2 cups low fat ricotta cheese	5 large eggs
Salt and coarse black pepper	Basil
1 cup Parmesan cheese	

Cover the bottom of your baking pan with a little olive oil, followed by the red sauce of your choosing. Bottled sauce: Newman's Tomato and Basil (regular, not the organic which has tomato paste in it) is fine. Sauce should cover the bottom of the pan, then place strips of uncooked rice, corn, or other gluten free lasagna noodles over them. While sometimes rice noodles get slimy on their own, in lasagna rice lasagna noodles seem to work well. There should be enough sauce to give the pasta fluid, but not enough for them to swim in.

Add a layer of the cheese mixture.

Then add another layer of lasagna noodle strips, then more sauce, then another layer of cheese mixture, then more noodles, and finally top with a sauce layer covered by fresh mozzarella and/or provolone cheese. Even people who aren't gluten free often prefer this type of lasagna. Garnish with fresh basil leaves before serving with a salad and GFbread.

Polenta Paradise

You can buy polenta in rolls the store, but homemade is better and not that difficult to make. Boil 6 cups water and add 2 cups yellow corn meal slowly, stirring constantly. Add salt and 1/4 cup butter. Then add Parmesan cheese into it. You can fry it in olive oil in a skillet and add tomato sauce and cheese on top. Or you can bake it with tomato sauce and cheese on top. You can add all kinds of vegetables and basil on it. Polenta is an incredibly flexible food that can be transformed and molded into a plethora of amazing dishes.

Knockout Noodle Kugel

This is a gluten free variation of an ethnic Eastern European dish that can be used as a main course or side dish. Boil 2 packages of corn noodles and add them to the following mixture:

1 cup sour cream	1 cup sugar
1 cup mozzarella cheese	1 Tablespoon cinnamon
1 cup cheddar	5 eggs
1 cup ricotta	1 Tablespoon vanilla

Put a stick of butter into a pan and let it melt. Then add the noodle mixture. This will make the edges crispy. Bake at 350 for 40 minutes. This recipe is good hot or cold, although I prefer it hot.

Gluten Free Gnocci

Boil 2 lb potatoes, then mash them.

Add them to 1 cup gluten free flour, 2 teaspoon salt, 1 egg, 1/2 cup melted butter, and some Parmesan cheese.

Make the mixture into a dough and then shape it into a cylinder or rope. Cut it into 1/2-inch bits. Drop them into salted water and boil them until done, Serve with sauce of your choice.

Indian Foods

Indian cuisine is easy to transform into gluten free menu items. Many gluten free premade sauces are available from major grocery store chains and they're delicious and easy to use.

Classy Curried Vegetables

The simplest is to open 3 cans of mixed vegetables and add to chicken or vegetable broth along with curry powder or gluten free curry sauce. Potatoes, carrots, and peas are the heart of any curry, so if the canned or frozen type you're using doesn't have enough of them, add a few more on your own. Of course, using your own fresh vegetables is best, but more time consuming.

You'll be able to find a large variety of gluten free curry powders and pastes. In general, go with the paste in the jar, and go for mild. The hot really is hot. While I love the heat, lots of people can't deal with it, and I find that spices are almost always hotter than I expect.

Let your curry simmer and make it as thick or runny as you want. Serve with white rice—jasmine is best.

Pleasing Pakoras

These are essentially fried vegetable fritters.

2/3 cup rice or tapioca flour	1/4 teaspoon baking soda
5 Tablespoons water	1/2 cup slivered onions
1/2 cup finely diced potato	2 cup oil
2 Tablespoons cilantro	

cumin, cayenne, salt, pepper, turmeric to taste

Mix vegetables, spices, gluten free flour, and water. Form into balls and cook in oil. Serve with chutney or sauces of your choice.

Countless Curries

Curries can be made in a variety of ways and they are all delicious. Common varieties include: vegetable curry, potato curry, curried garbanzo beans, or curried green beans, cauliflower, or virtually any vegetable. Curries may also be referred to by flavor, such as green, red, or yellow curry (green is generally the spiciest, followed by red and then yellow; green curry gets its color from cilantro and/or coriander root, red from red chiles, and yellow from tumeric/indian style curry powder). Panang curry is made with a peanut base and Massaman is made from dried spices.

For the basic curry, sauté your vegetables and meat slowly in a little olive oil, then add the sauce you wish to use. The sauce is the critical thing—you can make your own from fresh or dried ingredients/spices or buy them in paste or bottled form. The issue is what you think tastes best and how much work you want to do in the preparation. The bottled versions are the most expensive, but also the most convenient. The products exist—you simply have to play around with them to determine what you like. I can't advise you since Indian foods can become signature dishes for a chef. I have my own favorites and have adjusted the spices to meet the palates of those I serve. You need to do the same, but this isn't that hard and the rewards can be amazing!

Don't Dis the Dal!

Dal is regarded as a common person's food, and is quite delicious. Dal or yellow split peas are cooked with onions, cumin, coriander and become soft. They may be served with rice or breads. This is an inexpensive dish to make and something people absolutely love. Take your time cooking the legumes and let them simmer with the spices you choose so your dal will explode with flavor.

Yvonne M. Vissing, Ph.D.
Christopher Moore-Vissing, BA

Mexican Cuisine

Mexican food is typically regarded as the most gluten free friendly cuisine available, short of salads. However, ensuring gluten free safety can be a bit complicated.

Corn tortillas are fine, but things are not always what they seem. You need to read the ingredients list, because some corn tortillas are made with a corn and wheat flour mix. Only 100 percent corn tortillas are safe. The same applies to corn chips. A corn chip may contain flour or gluten products, or be spiced with products that warrant them unsafe. Even if the chips or tortillas were made gluten free, if they are cooked in oils that have been contaminated with gluten, they won't be acceptable to someone with gluten intolerance.

Sauces are also a concern if they contain glutened spices (like MSG) or tomato paste. I almost never use tomato paste, many are not GF. In general, the fresher the ingredients, the safer the sauces are likely to be. Sauces can be made quite delicious and safe, but if canned or pre-made, processed sauces are used, it is essential that the restaurant know what is in them.

When it comes to main course ingredients, the natural foods rule prevails. The more natural the food, the healthier for everyone; the more processed it is, the more chances of contamination. Meats cooked with just salt and pepper are safe; marinating the meat is often unsafe, and covering meats with spices or sauces must be done with absolute attention to ensure no contact with gluten.

Beans are usually fine if they're cooked plain; when they are made fancy, something might contain gluten. Likewise, rice on its own is always safe, and when cooked with natural ingredients it should be tasty and safe. But many processed rice products contain gluten, so be sure to check whether or not the ingredients are gluten free.

Nachos, tacos, enchiladas, and tostadas can all be made gluten free. However, sometimes they contain products that gluten intolerant people cannot handle. Don't take anything for granted, not even corn, beans, and rice. Dishes like Nachos should be acceptable if the chips are safe and real cheese is used. But often, not-real-cheese products are used, or sauces like queso are poured on, and many such products are thickened or spiced with products that contain gluten. These pose significant problems for people with gluten sensitivities.

Here are a few basic recipes for Mexican type food:

Spanish rice

Don't use boxed or packaged rice unless you're sure it's gluten free. Making your own is easy and inexpensive. Cook standard rice (white or brown, as you choose), add tomatoes, green peppers, red peppers, onions, and add cumin, cilantro, coriander, and chili powder to create an excellent rice. Sometimes I add fresh gluten free salsa if I am in a hurry, as this adds a more robust flavor. You can also add hot peppers to achieve the taste or spiciness you desire.

Beans

You can soak and make your own, seasoning them with salt, pepper or other safe spices as you wish. But the canned beans are so convenient and good that I find it hard to justify not using them unless I've got lots of time. Refried beans are usually safe and canned white, black, red, pink or pinto beans are too. You can doctor them up with fresh cilantro, onion, or top with cheese to make these flexible foods exactly as you want them.

Nachos

You can choose from a large variety of gluten free corn chips, or fry your own after cutting 100 percent corn tortillas into pieces. Make sure you've never used breaded or glutened items in your fryer. A mix of blue, red, and yellow corn chips will make your dish seem exotic.

The basic nacho topping is cheddar cheese or a combination of cheeses, such as muenster. After that, be creative. You can add green or red peppers, hot peppers, onion, or even zucchini, carrots, and other vegetables before (or after) popping the nachos into the oven.

You get to choose whether you cook the vegetables with the nachos or leave them crisp and fresh. Lettuce and guacamole should always be put on last. Some people like chicken or beef on their nachos for added protein, but this should be an al a carte item that people can choose for themselves. Never use mall or movie theatre type melty cheese; always use fresh grated cheese to avoid contamination issues.

Guacamole

Mash 2 ripe avocados and mix with fresh lemon or lime juice (personally I love the results with lime)

A little minced onion

Minced cilantro leaves

Diced tomatoes

Chopped green chilies and salt and pepper to taste

Serve on chips or as sides on Mexican dishes.

Amazing Enchilada Lasagna

Enchiladas are challenging gluten free dishes to make because of two issues—the sauce and the wrappers.

Sauce: I've searched for a canned or bottled gluten free enchilada sauce and haven't found "the one" yet. I end up making my own.

Fresh tomatoes, diced

Red and green peppers, cut in small pieces

Diced onion	Cilantro
Spicy V-8	Chili powder, cumin
Olive Oil	Lime juice
Corn starch	

In a skillet add the oil and saute the onion, then add the tomatoes and peppers. When soft, add the V-8 and spices. Slowly add corn starch to thicken the sauce a bit. Add the cilantro last.

Getting the right consistency right—thick enough but not too thick—is difficult because consumers are used to a flowing red sauce, not a chunky primavera sauce that resembles salsa. If you want a smooth sauce, all you have to do is put these ingredients into a food processor to liquefy the ingredients.

Filling: I love cheese enchiladas, especially if they have a little onion or green chilies added. Some people like meat fillings, or combine cheese, meats, and veggies. It's your choice. Cheese is a must; cheddar or a mix is recommended. The amount you use is up to you.

Construction: I no longer try to wrap cheese in corn shells to bake because, frankly, I can't get them to look pretty enough to resemble "normal" enchiladas." When I go out to eat, many restaurants seem to have products that enable them to do this, which is super. But I find the shells I buy tend to crumble and break while I'm folding them over. So I make enchilada lasagna, and here's how:

In a baking dish, place some olive oil on the bottom, then a layer of 100 percent fresh corn tortilla shells. Then add your filling and a little sauce, then another layer of tortilla shells, then another layer of filling, then the shells again, smothered by the sauce, and finally covered with more cheese before popping it into the oven. Served with a side of rice and beans, and a little guacamole, this dish is heavenly.

Quesadillas

Put a little oil in a skillet and add a fresh corn taco shell filled cheeses, meat or vegetables of your choosing. Place another shell on top, and when the bottom is golden crisp, flip it to brown the other side. Then enjoy your quesadillas, hot and delicious! Make more than you think you need because they will disappear fast!

Asian Cuisine

It seems that Chinese, Japanese, and other Asian culture foods would be gluten free, but take nothing for granted in the food world. Unadultrated rice is gluten free. Fresh vegetables used in most dishes are perfect. The chicken, beef, fish and pork start out fine. But soy sauce, marinades, and other sauces can be real problems, because they usually contain gluten related substances. We regularly use San J gluten free tamari sauce or products from Premier Japan or Green Valley Ranch. They make lovely sauces that are safe for gluten free diners. Having a good sauce is the key to fine cooking.

Rice crackers and products should be gluten free, but not if they've been treated with monosodiuim glutamate. I have a wok and tend to cook most of my Chinese and Japanese foods at home because the options available to us near where we live aren't good. Here are some of our favorite tried-and-true recipes:

Pad Thai

1 lb of thin rice noodles, cooked al dente.

2 Tablespoons peanut butter	5 Tablespoons gf soy sauce
1 Tablespoon brown sugar	2 scrambled eggs
6 scallions, diced	Peanuts

Paprika, chili powder, salt, pepper

1/4 to 1/2 cup cider vinegar

Bean sprouts

Cilantro leaves

Lemon or lime juice and wedges

Tofu or slender slices of sautéd chicken

Saute onions in peanut oil. Mix in soy sauce, sugar, peanut butter and spices with vinegar. Slowly add noodles and eggs, making sure to get the taste and consistency you like. Garnish with peanuts, fresh pea pods, fruit or cilantro. Sometimes I add crushed red pepper and toasted sesame seeds. This dish is awesome hot or cold.

Stir Fry Vegetables

If you have a wok, that's great. Otherwise a skillet works fine. Saute carrots, celery, green pepper, pea pods, bok choy, sprouts, broccoli, scallions, and whatever else you want in gluten free soy sauce or tamari or teriyaki sauce. Don't overcook them. You can add chicken, beef, or seafood. Garnish with cashews, almonds or peanuts. Serve with rice.

Sweet and Sour Chicken and Vegetables

Cook rice and set aside. In a skillet, sauté small pieces of chicken (bite size pieces) in a little oil. When the chicken turns a lovely brown color, add gluten free soy sauce and pineapple juice, either from a can or fresh. You may add a little orange juice if you must, but pineapple is best. Add in rice vinegar, salt and pepper. The amount of vinegar should be a bit less than the pineapple juice. Slowly mix in a little cornstarch, stirring well to make sure there are no lumps. The sauce should have substance, but not be too thick. Then add slices of green pepper, carrots, celery, and onion. When they just begin to turn a little less crunchy, add hunks of pineapple and stir well. Some people like to add pea pods, water chestnuts or bean sprouts, but these are a matter of choice. Adjust the sweet or sour (juice or vinegar) to please your palate. Remove from the heat and serve immediately over the rice. This is scrumptious.

Other Delightful Main Dishes

Spanakopita

Phyllo dough is the traditional base for this Greek dish, but there is no gluten free substitute at this time. I make it without the phyllo, using these ingredients:

2 lb fresh spinach	7 eggs
1/2 to1 lb feta cheese	1 onion sautéed in oil
Olive oil	Salt, pepper, oregano

Put spinach in a bowl filled with warm salt water to pull off any dirt. Then rinse and it will be ready to use. Sautee the onion in butter. Add the spinach and onion into the beaten egg and crumbled feta in a bowl, along with the spices. Butter the pan you plan to use. Pour into a well greased baking dish. You can create a gluten free, butter cracker crumb base if you want. Bake at 375 degrees for 40 minutes or until golden brown.

Shuggie's GF Quiche

Basic Recipe: Mix 1 cup plain yogurt with 6 eggs. Add cheddar cheese and a little parmesan cheese, along with some salt, pepper, and 2 Tablespoons gf flour. Mix well. Pour it into an uncooked GF pie shell and pop it into a 350 oven for a half hour. Throw potatoes in to bake for an easy, quick dinner (with a salad).

You can make all kinds of changes to the quiche: Add green peppers, tomatoes, and bacon for a Western quiche. Always cook zucchini first, before adding it to the quiche, and add cheeses to it. You can add onions and tomatoes for a French Provencal type quiche, olives and basil for Italian type, and so on.

Special Holiday GF Meatless Meat Loaf

This recipe was given to us by an elderly woman who babysat for us and we have modified it to be a staple in our gluten free holiday dining. Chop 1 onion sauteed in butter, add to 5 eggs, 30 oz cottage cheese, 1/2 cup grated or cubed cheddar cheese, 1/2 cups or more of chopped walnuts, dried onions, salt, pepper, a Tablespoon of A-1 and mix in 4 cups of gf Corn Flakes. Baked in greased pan at 350 degrees for an hour, covered, and 20 minutes uncovered. Let sit 5 minutes before cutting.

Ratatouille

This vegetable delight can be eaten alone, on gluten free pasta, risotto, rice, or with gf bread or crackers. A little Italian grated cheese on top makes it even better.

1 onion	1 eggplant
2 bell peppers	3 medium zucchini
1 cucumber	2 cloves garlic
4 Tablespoons olive oil	broth
5 tomatoes	

Sautee all the vegetables in the oil, then add the tomatoes and broth. Let it simmer slowly for a long time. This delicious dish can be served with pasta, risotto, or as a side to baked chicken. I like to put mozzarella cheese on top before I serve it.

Walnut Cheese Balls

This is another family favorite and we can't speak highly enough of the results. The dish is so elegant we like to use when cooking fine dining style.

1-1/2 cup walnuts	4 oz cheddar cheese
1/2 cups gf breadcrumbs	1/2 sauted onion
1/4 cup milk	2 Tablespoons parsley
2 eggs	pepper, salt
Bechemal sauce for the top.	

Mix the eggs, milk, gf breadcrumbs, cheese, onion, spices, and then add walnuts last. Form into balls with your hands. Put into well-greased pan and top with gf Bechemal sauce. Bake at 375 for half an hour or so.

Shuggie's Welsh Rarebit

There is no reason why someone who is gluten free should have to miss the most wonderful of foods! To us, Welsh rarebit is a comfort food that can easily be transformed for gluten free dining with two minor changes. Use GF flour instead of wheat flour in the sauce, and toast GF slices of bread instead of using wheat English muffins. We don't use beer in our recipe because we think it tastes richer and better with a milk base.

Melt 2-3 Tablespoons butter in a pan. Add 2 Tablespoons gluten free f flour to make a paste, and then add milk to smooth it out. Add 2 beaten eggs, some GF mustard (dry or wet), 1 Tablespoon Worcestershire sauce, and lots of sharp cheddar cheese. I always add some dry Parmesan cheese, as it give it a little salty taste and the consistency helps thicken the dish. If you like a spicy flavor, add some Cabot habenaro cheese.

Let it simmer until thick and lovely. Serve on toasted GF bread. If you have sauce left, it's easy to transform it into a cream soup of some sort. I usually use it with a potato, broccoli, or cream of cauliflower soup.

Sloppy Joes

Sloppy Joes are a delight, and as a base can be used in a variety of different foods. We use ground turkey browned in olive oil, fried with chopped onions, and add green pepper if you have any. When browned well, pour in Heinz Ketchup, a couple Tablespoons of French's mustard, and a dash of A-1 and Worcestershire sauce. Let it cook slowly and long. Serve on sandwiches with gluten free buns, baked potatoes, pasta, with Mexican food, and use leftovers in chili.

Breads

Bread is the most challenging of all the gluten free foods to cook, in my opinion. Yeasty wheat bread may be light and fluffy or wholesome and hearty, but gluten free breads tend to be on the heavy side, and as a result are challenging to bake in a way that produces an acceptable alternative to wheat bread. The closest I've come is by using King Arthur gluten free flour products. The closest pre-baked store bread is made by Udi's products, which are pretty fine when grilled.

A variety of bread mixes are available today, so I encourage you to try different brands and decide which you like best. Some breads make terrific muffins or fried breads instead of loaf types, while others resemble traditional bread when it bakes.

Gluten free Sandwich Bread

NOTE: King Arthur Flour has put their Gluten Free Sandwich Bread recipe online at <u>http://www.kingarthurflour.com/recipes/gluten-free-sandwich-bread-recipe</u>

Hands-on time:	14 mins. to 20 mins
Baking time:	38 mins. to 42 mins.
Total time:	Overnight, 2 hrs 37 mins. to 3 hrs 2 mins.

Ingredients

- 3 cups King Arthur Gluten Free Multi-purpose Flour or brown rice flour blend
- 3 Tablespoons sugar
- 2 teaspoons instant yeast
- 1-1/4 teaspoons salt
- 1-1/4 teaspoons xanthan gum
- 1 cup warm milk
- 4 Tablespoons soft butter
- 3 large eggs

Tips

- Like a baguette, this bread has a short shelf life. For best texture, reheat or toast after the first day.

- Make delicious cheese bread by reducing the sugar in the recipe to 1 Tablespoon and stirring 1 cup (4 ounces) shredded sharp cheddar cheese into the dough just before scooping it into the loaf pan.

- If you have a 9" x 4" x 4" pain de mie pan (Pullman loaf pan), this is a great time to use it. It will bake a taller loaf than a standard loaf pan. Bake with the lid on, or off. Baking with the lid off will give you a slightly more crowned loaf; leaving the lid on creates a slightly closer-grained loaf. If you use the lid, bake the bread for 50 minutes, with the lid on the whole time. Remove it from the oven, remove the lid, and turn it out of the pan onto a rack to cool.

- If you prefer to make this mix without eggs, using flax in place of the eggs works well. To replace the 3 eggs called for, use 1/4 cup plus 2 Tablespoons (1-1/2 ounces) flax meal (the more finely ground the better), blended with 1/2 cup plus 1 Tablespoon water. Let the mixture sit for 10 minutes to thicken before beating into the butter in the bowl. 1 egg recipe: 2 Tablespoons (1/2 ounce) flax meal (the more finely ground the better) blended with 3 Tablespoons water. Let it sit for 10 minutes to thicken before using.

- Note: For a dairy-free version of this bread, substitute margarine for the butter; and soy milk, almond milk, or rice milk for the milk called for in the recipe. Results may vary from the original.

Directions

Place the flour or flour blend, sugar, yeast, salt, and xanthan gum in a bowl, or the bowl of your stand mixer. Mix until combined. Using an electric mixer (hand mixer, or stand), drizzle in the milk, beating all the time. The mixture will be crumbly at first, but once all the milk is added, it'll come together. Add the butter and beat until thoroughly blended. Beat in the eggs one at a time, beating each in thoroughly before adding the next. Scrape the bottom and sides of the bowl, and then beat at high speed for 3 minutes, to make a very smooth, thick batter.

Cover the bowl, and let the thick batter rise for 1 hour. Scrape down the bottom and sides of the bowl, gently deflating the batter in the process. Grease an 8 1/2" by 4 1/2" loaf pan, or a 9" x 4" x 4" pain de mie pan (Pullman loaf pan). Scoop the dough into the pan. Press it level, using a spatula or your wet fingers. Cover with greased plastic wrap, and set in a warm place to rise until the loaf barely crowns above the rim of the 8 1/2" x 4 1/2" pan; or till it comes to within about an inch of the rim of the 9" pain de mie pan. This should take about 45 to 60 minutes. Toward the end of the rising time, preheat the oven to 350° F. Bake the bread for 38 to 42 minutes, until golden brown. If you're using a pain de mie pan, leave the lid on the entire time. Remove the bread from the oven, turn it out of the pan, and cool on a rack.

You Can Make Your Own Blend: Many gluten free recipes use our King Arthur Gluten Free Multi-purpose Flour, which includes ingredients that reduce the grittiness sometimes found in gluten free baked goods. This flour also increases the shelf life of your treats, keeping them stay fresh longer. The following make-at-home blend, featuring stabilized brown rice flour, works pretty well when substituted, and it tastes better than a blend using regular brown rice flour.

Whisk together 6 cups (32 ounces) King Arthur stabilized brown rice flour; 2 cups (10-3/4 ounces) potato starch; and 1 cup (4 ounces) tapioca flour or tapioca starch. Store airtight at room temperature. Note: You can substitute white rice flour for the brown rice flour if you like. Brown rice will make your baked goods grittier (unless you manage to find a finely ground version).

Desserts

Chris's Joe Frogger's

Here is Chris's favorite cookie. We have adapted it to be gluten free.

1/2 cup butter if you want them crispy
or Crisco if you want them chewy

1 cup white sugar	1 cup dark molasses
1/2 cup water	1-1/2 teaspoons salt
4 cups gluten free flour	1 teaspoons baking soda
1-1/2 t ginger	1/2 teaspoon cloves
1/4 teaspoons allspice	1/2 teaspoon nutmeg

Cream shortening and sugar. Mix in water and molasses. Sift in GF flour, salt, baking powder, spices. Cover and chill overnight. Preheat oven to 375. Lightly grease cookie sheets. Roll out cookie dough 1/4 inch thick on floured surface. Cut with round cookie cutter—3 inch type is recommended. Put on cookie sheets and sprinkle with additional sugar for topping. Bake 8–10 minutes. Leave cookies on sheet for 2-4 minutes to let them firm up before you take them off, or they may break.

Molton Fudge Brownies

2 ounces unsweetened chocolate

1 stick butter	1 cup sugar
2 eggs	1/2 cup gluten free flour

1/2 cup semisweet chocolate chips.

Bake in 8 x 8 pan at 375.

Do not bake more than 15 minutes or they will be overdone, which is a curse for good brownies. The secret in making delicious brownies is not to overcook them. You can even cook them even half-way, and make them more like hot fudge than cake. You determine how well you want them done, but don't overcook, because hard brownies are disappointing. If they turn out like molton lava they can be served hot under ice cream and taste heavenly.

Spiders

These original cult cookie/candies were made with chow mien noodles, but most of them contain barley, so cannot be used for gluten free diners. Here is our gluten free variety:

Thin gluten free pretzel sticks, snapped into halves

Large package of butterscotch bits

    (according to Celiac.com, Hershey and Kroger butterscotch bits are gluten free, but Nestle's are not).

Can of plain, salted, or unsalted peanuts

Melt butterscotch bits over slow fire (preferably in a double boiler). Add peanuts and pretzels. Don't add too many pretzels or the spiders will be dry and crumbly. Spoon mixture out onto wax paper so spiders can cool. As an alternative, gluten chocolate bits like Hershey's can be substituted for butterscotch bits.

Rice Krispie Treats

Tried and true, and always a favorite:

6 cups of gluten free Rice Krispies

1 ten-ounce package of marshmallows (40 regular, or 4 cups)

3 Tablespoons butter

Melt butter and marshmallows. Add Rice Krispies. Stir well. Pour into buttered pan. Cut into squares.

Celiac.com's Scotcheroos

1 cup sugar

6 cups gluten free Rice Krispies or Crispy Brown Rice

1 cup light corn syrup

1 cup gluten free semi-sweet chocolate chips

1 cup peanut butter

1 cup gluten free butterscotch chips*

Combine sugar and syrup in a 3 quart sauce pan. Bring to a boil, stirring constantly. Immediately remove from heat and stir in peanut butter. Add cereal and stir to coat cereal with mixture. Press into buttered 9 x 13 pan. Combine chocolate and butterscotch chips in medium microwave safe bowl. Microwave 1 minute, stir, and microwave 1 more minute. Stir until completely melted and well mixed. Spread evenly over cereal mixture in pan. Cool and cut into bars. *Hershey and Kroger brands are gluten free

No Bake Cookies

In pan, mix

2 cups sugar	1 cup butter or shortening
2 teaspoon vanilla	2 eggs
1 teaspoon salt	1 cup brown sugar
2-1/2 cups gluten free flour	1/2 cup sugar
1 teaspoon baking powder	1 stick butter
1-1/2 cup M & M candies or 1 cup choc	

Cook for 2 minutes.

Add 2-1/2 cups gluten free oats (Make sure they are certified GF, as regular oats usually aren't.), Quick oats set faster than whole oats, so adjust accordingly.

Add 1/2 cup gluten free peanut butter

1 tsp. vanilla

1/4 cup or more of cocoa

Take off heat and drop by spoonful onto wax paper. Cool and eat.

Edna's Peanut Butter Cookies

1/2 cup butter	1/2 cup white sugar
1/2 cup brown sugar	1/2 tsp. salt
1 egg	1/2 cup peanut butter
1/2 tsp. baking soda	
1-1/4 cup King Arthur Gluten Free Flour	

Blend butter, sugars, and salt. Add egg and peanut butter. Stir in flour and soda. Form balls the size of walnuts and place on greased cookie sheet. Press down with fork criss-crossed. Bake in 375 degree oven for 10 minutes.

PB Kiss Variation:

Mix ingredients above, then roll into balls. Roll each ball in white sugar. Bake for 3-5 minutes or so. Remove from hot over and place a Hershey's Kiss in the middle of the ball, pushing down slightly. Then put back into the oven for 2 minutes or until the kiss is warm but not melted. Remove from pan carefully and enjoy!

Chocolate Chip or M & M Cookies

Chocolate chip cookies and M & M cookies are both made with essentially the same batter. The only question is what you decide to put in at the end before baking.

1 cup butter or shortening	2 teaspoon vanilla
2 eggs	1 teaspoon salt
1 cup brown sugar	1/2 cup sugar
2-1/2 cups gluten free flour	1 teaspoon. baking powder

1-1/2 cup M & M candies or 1 cup chocolate chips.

Nuts like walnuts or pecans are always options.

Blend shortening and sugars in a large bowl. Beat in vanilla and eggs. Mix in dry ingredients. Stir in half the candies. Drop by teaspoons on ungreased cookie sheet. Decorate with remaining candy. Bake at 375 degrees for 10 minutes or until golden brown.

Butterscotch Brownies

1 cup brown sugar	1/3 cup butter
1 egg	3/4 cup gluten free flour
1 tsp. baking powder	1 teaspoon vanilla
1/2 cup nuts	Melt sugar and butter

Cool. Add remaining ingredients in saucepan. Spread in greased 11 x 7 pan for 350 degrees at 20 minutes.

Lemon Squares

Crust:

>1-1/2 cups gluten free flour,
>>favorites may be almond or coconut flour
>
>1 cup butter
>1/2 cup powdered sugar
>pinch of salt

Sift flour with sugar and salt. Cut in butter. Pat mixture into a 9 x 13 pan. Bake at 325 degrees until slightly brown, approximately 25 minutes.

Filling:

4 eggs	1-3/4 cup sugar

>6 Tablespoons fresh lemon juice
>4 Tablespoons gluten free flour or 3 Tablespoons cornstarch
>1/2 teaspoon baking powder

Beat eggs slightly and gradually add sugar. Stir in lemon juice, flour, and baking powder. Stir until smooth. Pour this mixture over baked crust while crust is still hot. Return to oven and bake for 25 minutes more. Remove from oven and sprinkle powdered sugar over pan while still warm. Cut in squares

GF Oatmeal Cookies

What's better than a warm oatmeal cookie with a glass of milk?

1-1/2 cup gluten free flour	1 teaspoon baking soda
1 teaspoon salt	1 cup butter
1 cup sugar	1 cup brown sugar
2 eggs	
2 cups certified gluten free oats	

Optional:

1 cup nuts, 1 cup chocolate chips, 1 cup GF butterscotch bits, or a dash of cinnamon

Cream sugar and eggs. Add dry ingredients. Stir in chocolate chips and nuts. Drop by teaspoons on cookie sheet. Bake 8 to 10 minutes at 350 degrees.

Joetta's Cherry Coconut Bars

1 cup gluten free flour	1/2 cup butter
3 Tablespoon powdered sugar	1/2 cup flaked coconut
2 eggs	1 cup sugar
1/4 teaspoon salt	1 teaspoon vanilla
1 cup maraschino cherries	Slivered almonds for top

Mix flour, powdered sugar and butter together and press into a greased 8 x 8 x 2 inch pan. Bake for 25 minutes at 350 degrees. Cool a little. Beat 2 eggs slightly, and stir in 1 cup sugar, 1/4 cup flour, 1/2 tsp. baking powder, 1/4 tsp. salt, 1 tsp. vanilla, 1/2 cup flaked coconut, and 1/2 cup (or more) maraschino cherries. Spread over pastry. Top with a few slivered almonds. Bake 20 minutes at 350 degrees. Cool and cut.

Haystacks

GF caramels – 1 bag
1 stick butter
1/2 cup sweetened condensed milk
Marshmallows
GF Rice Krispies

Melt 1 bag GF caramels, 1 stick butter, and 1/2 cup sweetened condensed milk over hot water in a double boiler. Coat marshmallows with mixture, and roll in gluten free Rice Krispies. Keep caramel mixture on hot water to keep thin enough to coat marshmallows. Cool before eating.

Seven Layer Bars

These are delicious and normally aren't gluten free because they're made with graham crackers. But it is easy to modify them to gluten free with this recipe.

1 stick butter, melted in 9 x 13 pan

Add in this order:

1 layer of gluten free cookie crumbs. (My favorite is to crush Pamela's Product Pecan shortbread or Enjoy Life's Vanilla Honey Graham cookies.)

1 layer of gluten free butterscotch bits

1 layer coconut

1 layer pecans or walnuts

1 layer chocolate chips

1 can Eagle brand milk, poured over top

Bake at 350 degrees until melted, about 15 minutes. Cut into hefty pieces, since most stores sell skimpy ones, and you will make friends for life.

Cheese Cake

Cheese cake is marvelous hot out of the oven, at room temperature, or cold out of the fridge.

Crust: Melt 1 stick of butter and mix with enough crumbs to cover the bottom or your pie pan or cheese cake bottom. For the crumbs, I recommend crushing GF shortbread cookies or even GF Oreo type cookies. You can add a handful of sugar and melted butter to help solidify the crust.

Filling:

2 bricks of cream cheese at room temperature

4-5 eggs   1 cup sugar

1 cup yogurt or sour cream

1/2 teaspoon baking powder

1 Tablespoon cornstarch

1 Tablespoon almond extract (or vanilla- but I think almond is a zillion times better in most dishes)

Mix together and pour into unbaked crust. Bake at 350 degrees for about 40 minutes or until it seems firm and light brown to the top. Don't let it over bake.

You can eat it warm or wait.

Variations: Serve it with fruit, whipped cream, or a variety of other toppings. Be creative. You can also mix in chocolate and swirl it into the batter for a swirled cheesecake. You can add ginger to the batter, or lemon rind. Each time you add an ingredient, stick with only one extra or the flavors may be too overwhelming. One of my favorites is to mix fresh raspberries into real whipped cream, top the cheese cake, and garnish with a raspberry and a mint leaf. OMG!

Persimmon Cookies or Pudding

Persimmons are common in the Midwest. Wild persimmons are small and sweet, hard to find. More likely in the fall you can find the large Japanese persimmons in stores. Their flavor isn't as fine but any persimmon is better than no persimmons for people who love them.

The base consists of:

1 cup persimmon pulp	1 cup sugar
1 teaspoon. baking soda	2 eggs
1/2 cup shortening or melted butter	
Cinnamon, nutmeg, cloves or ginger (don't add too much)	

Mix all these ingredients together.

To make persimmon pudding: Add 1-1/2 cup gluten free flour, 1 teaspoon baking powder, and raisins if you want. Pour into greased baking pan and put into oven for approximately a half hour at 350 degrees.

It is important to note that pudding can be of two forms: one is a firm bar, which is similar to Grandma Edna's recipe given above,

However, others like theirs to be looser in consistency, somewhat like Indian Pudding. If you prefer yours to be thinner to be eaten with a spoon, and perhaps ice cream or whip cream on top, then add milk, buttermilk or cream to the mixture.

To make persimmon cookies: Add 2 cups gluten free flour and add nuts or raisins if you like. Drop by teaspoonsful on a greased cookie sheet and bake for 10 to15 minutes at 350 degree oven.

Great Grandmother's Gingerbread Recipe

1/2 cup sugar	1 egg
1 cup hot water	1/2 cup butter and shortening mixed
1 cup molasses	2-1/2 cups sifted gluten free flour
1-1/2 teaspoon soda	1 teaspoon cinnamon
1 teaspoon ginger	1/2 teaspoon cloves
1/2 teaspoon salt	

Cream shortening and sugar. Add beaten eggs, molasses, then dry ingredients sifted together. Add hot water last and beat until smooth. Bake in greased shallow pan 35 minutes in moderate oven (325-250 degrees). This recipe is over 100 years old and modified for a gluten free diet.

Other Fine Recipes

Chocolate Shell for Ice Cream

One nice thing about going gluten free is that you start looking at ingredients, cost, and substitutions. Once this process begins, you'll find all kinds of ways to eat better, healthier, and for less money. Us New Englanders love ice cream and pouring chocolate shell on them is delicious. But most the products on the market are expensive and contain a list of ingredients with four-syllable words. As a nutritionist friend once said, "If a food has ingredients with more than three syllables, it's probably not healthy." So Chris found the following recipe, and now we can have healthy, affordable chocolate shell whenever we want.

2 Tablespoons coconut oil (fyi, this comes in a jar, not a bottle)

2 cups chocolate (your choice, just make sure the chocolate is gluten free. Hershey's is fine, Baker's chocolate can be, but other name-brand chocolates may not be. So don't assume just because a chocolate brand has a fancy name or costs a lot that it is safe).

Mix these two ingredients and put into the microwave, stirring. The results will be on the thin side. Poor it on to the ice cream and it hardens almost immediately. We store our leftovers in the fridge, and it is easy to microwave whenever we want to use it.

Barbeque Sauce

There are many delicious and safe barbeque sauces on the market. Are you grilling and you've run out of barbeque sauce? No problem! Just mix Heinz ketchup, French's mustard, and brown sugar together for a quick, safe, and cheap substitution. You can add some GF liquid smoke for variation, or add hot peppers to make it more like a chipotle sauce.

Yvonne M. Vissing, Ph.D.
Christopher Moore-Vissing, BA

A Note on Gluten Free Cooking

Being a gourmet gluten free cook means cooking healthy. It means:

- purchasing foods in their natural state as much as possible
- buying high quality food,
- cooking simply and letting the food's essence come out instead of masking the taste,
- cooking in a clean kitchen with clean equipment,
- appreciating the natural elegance of dining, and
- delighting in what you eat.

All this is to our benefit, no matter who you are or what kind of diet we wish to pursue.

Gluten free meals are good for everyone. Almost anyone can eat gluten free breakfasts, lunches and dinners, while traditional meals often contain nothing a gluten free diner can eat.

Shifting to a healthy-for-everyone cooking style isn't that hard, and you'll find it's cheaper in the long run. While we love to go eat out, I have a secret to tell you. Shhhhh. . . I'm the best cook I know. I was always a good cook, but going gluten free has made me even better. Sure, there are a few things I don't make anymore, and admittedly some dishes (like grain-based bread) that I miss. But seriously, now I pay more attention to what I'm fixing and how I fix it. We eat less volume and more quality.

I find it's easy to tweak old favorite recipes and turn them into new ones that are better for us. The most important thing is a willingness to change.

Cooking gluten free is

- Easy.
- Healthy.
- Affordable.
- Delicious.

What more could you want?

Chapter 7
Being Gluten Free

LIVING GLUTEN FREE can be easy, affordable, and delicious. It isn't a big deal once you know how to do it properly. By now, going GF is second-nature to us; we don't even think about it. We know how to cook, what to buy, where to shop, and the fine points of going out to eat. We have culinary confidence on how to cook gluten free in a way that fits into our busy lifestyles.

Chris is healthier since we went gluten free. And do you know what? So is the rest of our family. And you know what else? We're finding more and more people in our lives who have celiac disease. Food bonds people together—it always has and it always will.

The biggest obstacle to successful gluten free cooking occurs not in the kitchen, but in the brain. If you consider it a huge burden, that's how you'll live. But there is no reason to feel penalized because you have to go gluten free. Embrace this as an opportunity to live a healthier lifestyle. Our gluten free cooking has makes it harder for us to accept poor quality food and service when we dine out, because we're used to the best at home.

When we first started going gluten free, we weren't emotionally prepared to make the transition. Our mental resistance led to practical obstacles that made the foods less tasty. Trial and error helped smarten us up. Being willing to take risks was essential. Now we've learned to cook gluten free without cross-contamination. In our house, living with gluten and living gluten free are harmonious.

Once you get the hang of gluten free living, you'll learn to feed your family and friends delicious gluten free foods without stressing. You'll learn to have fun experimenting in the kitchen. Finding new recipes and sharing them is a loving way to bond with those we care about. Checking out places to go out to eat together need not be burdensome. Giving each other the food we need is an act of loving kindness.

For people in the food business, it's important to recognize that the gluten free consumer demographic is increasing exponentially. Their huge, active social network is adding new customers every day. Ignoring this group is sheer stupidity. For restaurants, the consequences of failing to address the needs of gluten free customers can lead to lost business and even lawsuits. Customers need to know if a restaurant is safe to patronize.

As you finish this book you will begin (or refine) your journey into gluten freedom. Embark on this adventure with zest and zeal.

Don't get taken by buying bad gluten free tasting products that cost too much.

Don't patronize places that are insensitive to your dietary needs.

Be honest and forthright about what you need.

We hope you'll check out the gluten free website we've shared with you in this book, and we'd love to hear from you. Learn, experiment, share, and be willing to fully engage with others in the gluten free community. We are a group of fascinating, fun, and flexible people. And we're damn good cooks.

You will love us, love the food, love your new life, and love going gluten free.

Happy dining!

Appendix
Special Assistance for Restaurants

FOR PEOPLE IN THE FOOD BUSINESS, many groups are ready and willing to help with gluten free dining. Here is a partial list:

The Gluten free Restaurant Awareness Program (GFRAP)

The GFRAP (http://www.gluten.net/gfrap/) facilitates the relationship between restaurants and people who have celiac disease and other forms of gluten intolerance and helps build a win-win opportunity for restaurants to provide service to these people and gain increased patronage. Participating restaurants are able to provide gluten free meals from their regular meals. The GFRAP is a program of the Gluten Intolerance Group of North America. Participating GFRAP restaurants enthusiastically welcome gluten free diners. On this site you will find links, directions, and other valuable information about each participating restaurant. By working together, using consistent guidelines, and listing participating restaurants on one website, they are creating a network that allows people to socialize and travel with more confidence in dining away from home.

The Gluten free Food Service (GFFS) Accreditation Program

The GFFS (http://www.gffoodservice.org/) enables restaurants and other established food preparers to put the GFFS logo on advertising materials so patrons can verify the quality, integrity, and purity of that establishment's food preparation policies. It also ensures that the restaurant or food preparer has met certain education, policies and standards to be gluten free. The Gluten free Food Service Training and Management Accreditation Program is a GIG Industrial Program designed to work with food service establishments of all types who are serving, or want to serve, gluten free consumers.

GFRAP has developed a three point best practices formula to maintain the safety of gluten free food production and service. These include:

Principle 1: Prevention of food safety hazards is favored over reliance on corrective actions after a problem has occurred.

Principle 2: Prevention of food contamination in the production of gluten free foods must encompass all aspects of procurement, processing, and delivery of gluten free foods.

Principle 3: Worker hygiene and production and storage area sanitation practices play a critical role in minimizing the potential for contamination of gluten free foods.

This organization provides posters for the kitchen that offer quick reminders of what ingredients are safe or unsafe. They offer educational resources for restaurants. Many organizations find that being credentialed helps promote business.

Gluten free Education and Awareness Training (GREAT)

The National Foundation for Celiac Awareness has developed an online education and training program at http://www.celiaccentral. org/great-gluten free-foodservice-training/. The program provides power points and educational materials to help both individuals and food preparers address the needs of people who need gluten free foods. The training is also designed to help dietitians and health care professionals learn more about celiac disease and nutrition. Continuing education credit from the American Culinary Federation and the American Dietetic Association can be provided for some of their courses.

This group offers a 90 minute course designed to teach the essentials of gluten free safety from fridge to fork. It explains celiac disease and the gluten free diet, how to find gluten free foods and store them, safety protocols, how to avoid cross contamination, and how to successfully interact with gluten free customers. They provide:

Self-training, where students learn core competencies for gluten free preparation and serving. A training manual, syllabus, webinar presentation, competency exam, and certificate of completion are provided for this level of training.

Staff-Training, where restaurants receive a GREAT Kitchens Toolkit to train kitchen staff and workers in the dining room who interact with customers. A manual, a CD with training materials, a DVD, a window decal, and public relations tools are provided. Onsite training with a GREAT Kitchens instructor is available.

Celiebo Certification

Celiebo.com offers certification for restaurants so that both the restaurant and the customers know the food will meet the needs of gluten free diners. Their web address is http://www.celiebo.com/restaurants/.

This group helps restaurant owners make money by "serving the largest growing and most underserved community in restaurant dining." A restaurant's certification can be promoted through social media to let potential consumers know they understand the issues and make appropriate accommodations for customers who need a gluten free diet. They allege that certification will help ease management worries, knowing that an established protocol is in place within the restaurant. Chefs can be freed to reinvent their signature dishes as gluten free and take pride in creating dishes that gluten free customers enjoy.

The certification team comes to each restaurant and inspects the kitchen to make sure it meets standards to adequately prepare gluten free foods. Their team will train the staff on how to prepare and create a successful gluten free dining experience from A to Z. They provide educational materials as well as gluten free promotional materials.

Quality Assurance International Gluten free Certification Program

The Quality Assurance International Gluten free Certification Program is a part of a company called NSF International, which has been focusing on verification of food safety and public health practices for over 65 years and over 20 years of organic certification experience. Its website can be found at http://www.qai-inc.com/resources/gluten free program.asp

The QAI Gluten free Certification program is appropriate for food producers and manufacturers of gluten free products and attempts to verify the safe production, storage, and transport of gluten free products. It helps organizations avoid cross-contamination and provides a science based, third party verification process to ensure that organizations are gluten free. The certification program includes testing procedures, auditing processes, on-site annual inspections, and an independent application review process.

The Gluten free Certification Organization (GFCO)

The Gluten free Certification Organization (http://www.gfco.org/) is a program of The Gluten Intolerance Group®, also known as GIG®. This independent food processing inspection program verifies that food products meet the highest standards for gluten free ingredients and a safe processing environment. GFCO's scientific and professional board reviews their practices. GFCO inspects products for gluten and does not certify products for any other potential allergens. Foods that meet these standards receive a gluten free certification mark so consumers can easily identify foods that are free of gluten and cross contamination. The GFCO reviews ingredients and conducts onsite inspections.

Overview of How to be a Gluten Free Establishment

Here is a quick check-list of the recommendations made in this book.

1. Make a commitment to gluten free dining as part of your business.

2. Learn why gluten free dining is an important issue and convey this to your staff. This includes:

   - Health issues for people with celiac disease or gluten intolerance.

   - Problems these patrons face when dining out.

   - How these problems can be prevented in your establishment.

   - Why doing this is good business.

3. Become a part of organizations to support your move toward gluten free dining. These include:

   - The Gluten free Restaurant Awareness Program (GFRAP) http://www.gluten.net/gfrap/

   - The Gluten free Certification Organization (GFCO), http://www.gfco.org/

   - The Gluten free Food Service (GFFS) accreditation program (http://www.gffoodservice.org/)

   - The Gluten free Registry: http://glutenfreeregistry. com/

   - A Gluten free Guide to Restaurants: http://aglutenfreeguide.com/restaurants

- National Association of Catering Executives
  http://www.nace.net/
- Join other organizations or listings to learn, network, and share with others to promote your business and learn from them.
- Review key websites like Celiac.com periodically for education, information, resources, and news.

4. Review and alter your menu offerings.
   - Make sure you have good dining options for gluten free patrons.
   - See how you can modify existing menu options to make them safer and healthier for all patrons.
   - Create new menu options when necessary.

5. Consider your shopping strategies and options.
   - Do your suppliers carry gluten free foods?
   - What additional foods do you need to build your gluten free food staple base?
   - Where will you buy them locally? Identify your options.
   - Where can you buy them online? Identify your resources.

6. Scrutinize your kitchen hardware.
   - Make sure your pans, utensils, equipment, and cooking areas meet standards for safety.
   - Reduce contamination possibilities.

7. Evaluate your kitchen processes.
   - Review your training procedures.
   - Create standards, policies, and protocols to ensure safety and satisfaction.
   - Monitor and enforce them.
   - Alter as necessary.

8. Educate your wait staff.
   - Provide training opportunities, specifically addressing the need for allergen and gluten free services.
   - Monitor staff compliance.
   - Provide additional training and supervision.

9. Communicate effectively
   - Make gluten free dining options clear on your menu and website.
   - Train staff how to respectfully communicate with patrons regarding their dietary needs.
   - Communicate with chef and kitchen staff so they are aware of particular needs.
   - Talk with customers about what the kitchen can or cannot do, to accommodate their needs.
   - Check in with kitchen staff to make sure each order is prepared appropriately.
   - Serve the dishes well, without possibility of contamination.
   - Make sure each dish is satisfactory.
   - Provide training opportunities, specifically addressing the need for allergen and gluten free services.
   - Monitor staff compliance.
   - Check with your customers patron to ensure satisfaction.

10. Develop social networking to promote your menu options and sensitivity to gluten free dining
    - Facebook
    - Twitter
    - Restaurant webpage with menu options and link to allergy information for your dishes
    - Blogs
    - Testimonials
    - Email notices to patrons
    - Newspaper, TV, and radio articles about your gluten free dining options
    - Advertisements on TV, radio, and newspapers
    - Restaurant notices, cards, flyers on cuisine options
    - Provide information and support to local health organizations.
    - Participate in local health events, fairs, and conferences.

- Do periodic gluten food sample give-aways—the best way to convince people that gluten free foods are tasty and good for them.
- Consider supporting gluten free groups or sponsoring local gf groups.
- Be creative with getting the word out there.

Food providers who master these ten steps will meet the needs of an ever-increasing customer base who will become loyal fans and help the business grow. The ten steps are wise for dealing with any guest, so ultimately a food provider won't go wrong by implementing them—and may end up doing very well indeed.

Gluten free expertise should be an important component of any restaurant or kitchen. In this book, we provide the rationale, strategies, and resources anyone can successfully use to create delicious foods for gluten free diners. Restaurant owners and food preparers should also realize that the numbers of gluten free patrons will only continue to increase. It's time to get on board and move forward in this new direction, or risk being left behind at the station. Few restaurants want to wave goodbye to a lucrative component of their business.

At this point, many restaurants still assume a caveat emptor attitude: "Let the patrons beware of gluten on our menu." They may feel they're off the hook if a consumer doesn't tell the server they have a gluten sensitivity or they're silly enough to order something that isn't safe for them. But this attitude is going bye-bye. Gluten free consumers are demanding their rights to have a selection of foods from which to choose when they go out to eat. They have a right to know these foods are safe. They have a right to know what foods contain. They have a right to be served in a professional, respectful, and conscientious manner. They have a right to expect their foods will be served in a timely manner, and offered at a fair price.

If a food serving establish fails to address their rights, the one who loses in the long run is not the patron, who will simply go somewhere else next time (and tell their friends about their unpleasant dining experience). The big loser is you, the food provider. Word will spread quickly. It isn't just the gluten free patron you have to worry about, but their friends, family members, work colleagues, and anyone else they know.

We have eaten out at many places and can tell when a cook is inexperienced in gluten free cooking or when they have it down. Honestly, gluten free cooking is easy once you get the hang of it. That's why restaurant owners, kitchen managers, and cooks should be encouraged to learn the art of gluten free cooking.

We are happy to help provide anyone with the A to Z overview of how to make gluten free cooking easy and delicious. As consultants, we can help with menu preparation, shopping guides, kitchen instruction, serving styles, and communication with patrons. We recommend that restaurants engage in some of these training programs and receive official certification as gluten free establishment. This will help ensure that the staff continues to meet the safety standards of gluten free cooking.

Gluten free dining is not a fad. Gluten free is here to stay. Take a lesson from the fast food chain Subway, which decided to offer gluten free food in order for them to stay competitive in the marketplace. They spent three years developing gluten free sub rolls and brownies. They wanted products that tasted good, they could be proud of, and that customers would like. This they accomplished.

But they found that training employees to do things in a different way was challenging (AllergyEats.com 2011). At Subway, when a customer orders a gluten free roll or brownie, the line staff is required to wipe down the entire counter and get rid of any crumbs in the vicinity. Then they wash their hands and change their gloves. Gluten free rolls and brownies are pre-packaged on fresh deli paper. A single-use, pre-packaged knife is included for cutting so there will be no cross-contamination. The gluten free sandwich is taken from order to point-of-sale by the same person, instead of being passed down the line in the traditional Subway manner. Customers can watch the entire process from start to finish. They have firsthand knowledge assurance that the food they order will indeed be gluten free and safe from contamination. Staff members are trained to treat the gluten free customer the same way anyone would be treated, but with a little extra assurance to let them know the staff has taken all due safeguards in preparing their food.

We hope this information helps you!

References

Shana James Ahern. *Gluten Free Girl and the Chef.* (New York: Wiley, 2010).

Allergy Eats. "Subway Expanding Gluten Free Test." 2011. http://bit.ly/1BlJvQX

Amanda Baltazar. "Creating Loyal Customers." *Restaurant Management.* 2011. http://bit.ly/1KuJtbT

Mark Brandau. "US restaurant count continues to fall: Independents closed the most." *Restaurant News.* July 20, 2010. http://bit.ly/1D1VHrQ

Livia Borghese. "Italian scientists on trial over L'Aquila earthquake." *CNN.* 2011. http://cnn.it/18QTyEr

California Requirements for a Gluten free Commercial Kitchen. eHow.com last accessed December 12, 2013. http://bit.ly/1DIWUmq

Rachel Carson. Silent Spring. (Boston: Houghton Mifflin, 1962).

T. J. Carter and T. Gilovich. "The relative relativity of material and experiential purchases." *Journal of Personality and Social Psychology,* 98,1. (2010): 146-159.

"Celiac disease." Accessed January 6, 2015 at www.celiac.com.

P. Cureton. "Gluten free dining out – is it safe?" *Practical Gastroenterology.* November. (2006): 61-68.

Sam Dean, Sam. "How a bad rye crop may have caused the Salem witch trials." *Bon Appetit.* Oct. 17 (2012). http://bit.ly/1vutLfm

Jay Dwivedi "How to improve customer service." *I proceed.* Retrieved November 7, 2011. http://bit.ly/1uewSY5

Kyle Eslick. "McDonalds Gluten free Menu". Retrieved October 14, 2014. http://bit.ly/1AvTuWj

Alessio Fasano. *Gluten Freedom.* (New York:Wiley Publishers:2010).

Alessio Fasano, et al. "Prevalence of celiac disease in at-risk and not-at-risk groups in the United States." *Archives of Internal Medicine.* 163,3(2003):268–292.

Tom Feltstein. "A Fundamental Focus on Driving Sales is More Crucial than Ever." *Nation's Restaurant News.* April 6,43,12 (2009): 18.

Kasara Ferasat. "Five Tactics to Create A Sustainable Restaurant Business." *Graziadico Business Review.* 2010. Retrieved June 2, 2013. http://bit.ly/1zccr9J

Food Allergy and Anaphylaxis Network. *"Welcoming Guests with Food Allergies: A Comprehensive Program for Training Staff to Safely Prepare and Serve Food to Guests Who Have Food Allergies,* Food Allergy and Anaphylaxis Network [FAAN]". *Food Allergy and Anaphylaxis Network.* (2008): 1–58.

Gluten Free Easily. "50+ GF FOODS YOU CAN EAT TODAY!" (2009). http://bit.ly/1zjXWp1

Gluten Free Easily. "The GFE Pantry." (2009). http://bit.ly/1KuS2n2

Peter Green and Rory Jones. *Celiac Disease.* (New York: William Morrow: 2010).

Caroline Hadley. "Food allergies on the rise?" *Nature. EMBP Reports.*7 (2006):1080 - 1083 http://bit.ly/1ueDoOx

Marlys Harris. "Tricks of the Restaurant.7 Ways Menus Make You Spend." *CBS Money Watch.* Apr 17. (2011). http://bit.ly/1DJ6zsX

Healthy Villi. "Newly Diagnosed Workshop". (2014). http://healthyvilli.org

Ron Hoggan. "Top 20 Things You Should Know About the Impact of Gluten". Retrieved March 17 (2014). http://bit.ly/1CxZPRB

T. J. Jaccobberger. "Restaurants and social media: What works and what doesn't." *Inside Scoops.* Retreived March 16, 2013. http://bit.ly/1BXuMt9

Keeping It Kleen. "Prepping food properly: How to keep your kitchen clean." (2011). www.keepingitkleen.com

Maria Keller. "Safe Gluten Free Travel." *Today's Dietitian.* 13, 8 (2011): 14. http://bit.ly/1ueFMVo

Gina Kolata. "Doubt is cast on many reports of food allergies." *New York Times.* May 11. (2010). http://nyti.ms/1zTXXlS

G. Kristjansson et al. "Adverse reactions to food and food allergy in young children in Iceland and Sweden." *Scand J Prim Health Care* 17 (2010): 30–34.

Christine Lafavee, "Higher Learning, Higher Dining," *Restaurants and Institutions.* November (2007): 89–90.

Nancy Lapid. "What is gluten cross contamination and why should you worry about it? " About.com retrieved Feb. 5, 2015. http://abt.cm/1rq71aY

Ann Lee and Jackie Newman. "Celiac Diet: It's impact on quality of life." *Journal of the American Dietetic Association.* Nov. 103:11 (2003): 1533-5. http://bit.ly/16GLXaz

Living Strong.com. "Kitchen basics on gluten free cooking." Retrieved Feb. 2, 2015. http://bit.ly/1v1FxIy

J. Lowell. *Against the Grain.* (New York: Henry Holt and Co: 1995).

Deborah Manners. "Food Intolerance Symptoms, Food Allergies, and Food Insensitivity." Retrieved December 18 (2014). http://www.foodintol.com/

John McKean. *Customers Are People: The Human Touch.* (New York: Wiley: 2003).

Mindbiz.com. "How to make money in a restaurant." Retrieved December 28, 2013. http://bit.ly/1Kj49W7

Paul Mitchell. "You will retain more customers by meeting their emotional needs." *EZine.* http://bit.ly/16uZD81

John Moore. "Restaurant too successful for social media?" *Social Media Restaurant.* (2011). http://socialmediarestaurant.com/

Marion Nestle. *Food Politics.* (Oakland: University of California Press:2013). http://www.foodpolitics.com/

Ed O'Boyle. "Luring Customers Back." *Gallup Management Journal.* (2011). http://bit.ly/1vuDvGD

Elizabeth Olson. "Restaurants reach customers through social media." *New York Times.* 1,20 (2011) http://nyti.ms/16kVVNU

Bryan Pearson. *The Loyalty Leap: Turning Customer Information into Customer Intimacy.* (2011). http://pearson4loyalty.com/

B. Pereira et al. "Prevalence of sensitization to food allergens, reported adverse reaction to foods, food avoidance, and food hypersensitivity among teenagers." *J Allergy Clin Immunol* 116(2005): 884–892.

Amy Ratner. "Show me the Gluten free Money." Jan 6 (2011). http://bit.ly/1zDejfg

Ron Ruggless. "Restaurant Social Media: Looking for the ROI". *Restaurant News.* (2011). http://bit.ly/1D2jDv1

Michael Sansonl. "State of the Industry 2009: Survival Mode." *Restaurant Hospitality* February 26 (2009): 28-30.

Rick Saporito. "How to improve dining room service." (2011) http://bit.ly/1CybWOD

S. H. Sichere, S. S. Noone SA and A. Munoz-Furlong. "The impact of childhood food allergy on the quality of life." *Ann Allergy Asthma Immunol* 87,6 (2001): 461-4.

Allison St. Sure. "A brief history of wheat and why it is making us sick." *Sure Foods Living.* Sept 27 (2010). http://bit.ly/1C3jRAN

Allison St. Sure. "The emotions of dining out gluten free." Sure Foods Living. June **15 (2011)** http://bit.ly/1EJnKyc

Allison St. Sure. "Halloween Candy List Gluten free Allergen-Free 2014." Sure Foods Living. http://bit.ly/1rLejDU

Allison St. Sure. "Fibromyalgia, Chronic Fatigue and Gluten Intolerance." Sure Foods Living. http://bit.ly/1BXLNU3

Sam Taute. " Live from Fancy Food: How to improve your gluten free menu offerings." Smart Blog on Restaurants. Retrieved January 19, 2015. http://bit.ly/16v79Q8

T. Thompson. "Gluten contamination of commercial oat products in the United States." *New England Journal of Medicine*. 351 (2004): 2021-2022.

"U.S. Foodservice Industry Forecast," *Technomic, Inc.*, May 2009, http://www.technomic.com/facts/forecast.html.

L. Van Boven and T. Gilovich. "To do or to have? That is the question." *Journal of Personality and Social Psychology*, 85, 6 (2003): 1193-1202.

"Vegetarian Times Study Shows 7.3 Million Americans Are Vegetarians and an additional 22.8 Million Follow a Vegetarian-Inclined Diet." Retrieved December 28 2015. http://bit.ly/1uf98TM

Yvonne Vissing. Introduction to Sociology. (San Diego, CA: Bridgepoint Education: 2011).

Michael Young. *The Peanut Allergy Answer Book*. (Gloucester: Fair Winds Press, 2006).

M. Zarkadas and S. Case. "The impact of a gluten free diet on adults with Coeliac disease: Results of a national survey." *Journal of Human Nutrition and Dietetics*. 10, 1 (2006): 41-9.

We also wish to credit the many organizations and websites we have used throughout this book. We thank them for helping educate all of us about the many different aspects of gluten intolerance and how to dine more successfully.

Acknowledgements

We wish to thank all those who made our learning about celiac disease and going gluten free easier. This especially includes Judy Hill, who first made Chris aware of celiac disease running in the family and Daniel Leffler, MD, whose medical expertise dealing with gluten issues and health-related conditions has helped us and thousands of other people feel better. Thanks are given to Jessica Labun Placy, who showed us how good friends can go out of their way to make sure going gluten free is no big deal. We deeply appreciate how she learned to make beautiful and delicious gluten free foods for us. Learning how to be good cooks is a family tradition, so we want to acknowledge how Great-Grandma Grace and Grandma Edna understood that healthy foods were essential, and cooking them well was equally important.

We are greatly appreciative of the wisdom and assistance of Sammie Justesen, who understood the importance of this topic and helped craft it into the lovely book you are reading. And thanks to all of you who work in restaurants or stores and take the time to understand how important gluten freedom is for all the people who pass through your doors.

About the Authors

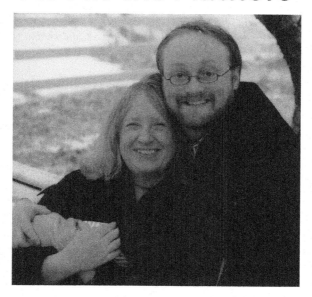

Yvonne Vissing, Ph.D., is the parent of three wonderful children and Professor of Sociology at Salem State University where she also is the founding director of its Center for Childhood & Youth Studies. A former National Institute of Mental Health Post-Doctoral Research Fellow and medical sociologist, she focuses on mind-body-society interrelationships.

Christopher Moore-Vissing, BA, is an independent film maker in New Hampshire. In addition to his love of film, his passions also include history, mental health, trivia, social media, and his old English bulldog, Magnus.

Yvonne M. Vissing, Ph.D.
Christopher Moore-Vissing, BA

Previous Publications by Yvonne M. Vissing

Books

Vissing, Y. *Introduction to Sociology.* Bridgepoint Publishing, CA. *2011.*

Vissing, Y. *How To Keep Your Children Safer: A Guide For Parents.* University of New England Press. 2006.

Vissing, Y. *Women Without Children: Nurturing Lives.* Rutgers University Press. June 2002.

Vissing, Y. and Peer, S. *Finding Information About Children: A Resource Guide to Using the Internet.* Nova Press. 2001.

Vissing, Y. *Out of Sight, Out of Mind: Homeless Children and Families in Small Town America.* University of Kentucky Press. 1996.

Chapters

Vissing, Y. Poverty and Homelessness: Impact on Educators. Conference Proceedings: The Invisible Child: Poverty in the Heartland. Rutgers University Press. NJ. 2005.

Vissing, Y. Researching Homeless Children. Research Issues in the Study of Children. Amy Best, editor. Sage Publishers. 2004.

Vissing, Y. Two entries in The Encyclopedia of New England Culture. One on housing policy, and one on homelessness. 2004.

Vissing. Y. Homelessness is a Problem in Rural Areas. In The Homeless: Opposing Viewpoints. Greenhaven Press. 2001.

Vissing, Y. Homelessness in Middle School Students. The Prevention Researcher. 2001.

Vissing, Y. "Meeting the Educational Needs of Intermediate and Middle School Homeless Students", in James Strong and Evelyn Reed-Victor's book, Promising Practices in Educating Homeless Students. Sage Publications. 2000.

Vissing, Y.M. and W. Baily. "Parent-to-Child Verbal Aggression" in Dudly Cahn and Sally Lloyd's forthcoming book, Communication and Family Violence. 1998. Sage Publications.

Hafferty, F., J. and Y. Vissing. "Professional Roles and Health Behavior" in David Gochman's book, Professional Behavior in Medicine. Sage. 1997.

Vissing, Y. "Heroic Students" in Cultural Diversity in Education, Sage, 1998.

Vissing, Yvonne and David Kallen. "The Clinical Sociologist in Medical Settings" in Handbook of Clinical Sociology. Howard Rebach and John Bruhn, eds. Plenum Publishing Co. 1990.

Index

Going Gluten Free

CPSIA information can be obtained at www.ICGtesting.com
Printed in the USA
BVOW08s0447090615

403746BV00002B/29/P